D0404357

"*Hug Therapy* disrupts the simple act of a hug, turning it into a way to spark connection within you, your community, with strangers…and it may just end up bringing our planet to awareness of being one. Crazy, awesome hugs—of course you should become a part of this movement!"

—Mich Hancock, cofounder of TEDxGatewayArch, Host of *MichMash* Podcast

"I'm excited to say I have now completed my 21-Day Hugging Journey. I found it powerful and useful. Stone has created a deceptively simple sounding twenty-one-day challenge that is in fact a *genius concept* when you understand how all the pieces he brings to it fit and work together. I have started to view each day differently in terms of how I interact with the people in my life. We can't get enough kindness and caring in the world. I am now starting to see how improvements with friends and family could ripple out to people in my neighborhood and much further into the world."

—Brian Lunt, Medici cofounder, inspiration behind Top-50 STL

"Before I was introduced to the twenty-one-day hugging challenge, I was depressed, anxious, and struggling with fibromyalgia. It wouldn't be too strong to say that I felt ready to nosedive into the pavement. Believe it or not, seven days after going on the

21-Day Hugging Journey on Facebook Live and reading *Hug Therapy*, I felt like a new man. I chronicled it all on Facebook and I would love for you to check it out. My life was transformed. I felt supercharged—no, wait—I *am* supercharged. I believe it's not a journey; it's a lifestyle. The biggest takeaway for me from the book was being radically transparent in everything I do. It totally freed me up to do greater good and be inspired in the process. I was made for this. Come with us on this journey. It meets you where you are, and you can create whatever really matters to you!"

—Gary Havel Jr. mailman, war hero, and hugging ambassador

"Dr. Stone has taken us far beyond the everyday hug. With his 21-Second hug, virtual hug, and 'space of a hug,' he invites us on a 21-Day Hugging Journey of discovery that opens up a whole universe of new windows into empathy, sharing, transforming, building community, and deeply *being* with other humans. So, if you see people walking down the street stopping for conversation, asking permission, breaking out into spontaneous, longer hugs, you will know that they have been reading this engaging, surprising, concise, and thought-provoking book. Join the fun and take the personal challenges. Get this book today. You just might see yourself and encounter others in a new, beautiful way."

—Lou Agosta, faculty member, Illinois School of Professional Psychology, and author of *A Rumor of Empathy*

HUG THERAPY

HUG THERAPY

A 21-Day Journey
to Embracing Yourself,
Your Life, and Everyone
Around You

Dr. Stone Kraushaar

CORAL GABLES, FL

Published by Mango Publishing Group, a division of Mango Media Inc.

Cover Design: Morgane Leoni
Layout & Design: Morgane Leoni

For permission requests, please contact the publisher at:

Mango Publishing Group
2850 S Douglas Road, 2nd Floor
Coral Gables, FL 33134 USA
info@mango.bz

For special orders, quantity sales, course adoptions and corporate sales, please email the publisher at sales@mango.bz. For trade and wholesale sales, please contact Ingram Publisher Services at customer.service@ingramcontent.com or +1.800.509.4887.

Hug Therapy: A 21-Day Journey to Embracing Yourself, Your Life, and Everyone Around You

Library of Congress Cataloging-in-Publication number: 2019941764
ISBN: (print) 978-1-64250-070-7, (ebook) 978-1-64250-071-4
BISAC: PSY031000—PSYCHOLOGY / Social Psychology

Printed in the United States of America

Please note that Hug Therapy, The Hug Doctor, and National Hugging Day are all trademarked.

Hug Therapy is dedicated to my mother Judy, whom I lost to cancer when I was twenty-five and she was fifty-two. Every hug I had with her was so precious and I didn't even realize how important they were.

"Your vision will become clear only when you can look into your own heart. Who looks outside, dreams; who looks inside, awakes."

–Carl Jung

Contents

Foreword

Dr. Stone and I share a wonderful distinction: we are both professional huggers. A hug is powerful and has the ability to turn every interaction into an opportunity for achieving profound richness. I chose the word *richness* instead of another word you might have expected—riches. Some of the richest people I've met are really the most deprived, because their financial abundance spotlights the lack of love and connection they feel. On the other hand, simple people who love and support each other often forget their financial lack in favor of a deeper, richer abundance—one where hugs are natural, welcomed, and often transformative.

When I heard about this amazing book, I practically jumped out of my seat. The benefits of this simple practice are at last being extolled by a man who not only appreciates its power, but has been personally transformed by it. Who other than "The Hug Doctor"™ and founder of Hug Therapy™ could have written it, and in a way that can benefit anyone? The stories, insights, and tools Dr. Stone shares help us see ourselves and the ways we've either neglected the simple power of hugging or welcomed it. When was the last time you walked up to a stranger and asked if they needed a hug? If you've ever taken such a risk, you likely discovered something interesting—that a good number of the people you ask will accept your offer.

And who knows where a single, meaningful hug might lead, especially for someone who feels disconnected or isolated. A warm hug just might change the world!

I've had the chance to travel to many of the world's biggest hotspots, and I didn't hold back the hugs. i remember when I visited Iraq for the first time in 1998. The country was isolated from the rest of the world, and welcoming an American Peace Troubadour seemed an unlikely solution. What did I do? I hugged as many people as I could, and though custom required I limit my hugs to men, even that rule was broken several times when it felt appropriate. The people I embraced lit up and accepted my affection, though I'm sure it was a great surprise for most of them. By the time I left Iraq, a true bond had been created with many of the people I met, and I wouldn't be surprised if that bond rippled through the streets of Baghdad.

The power of a hug was shown to me again not long after apartheid ended in South Africa. I was invited to meet with the leaders of several gangs running the streets of Cape Town. From the beginning, I wondered what I would say to them—what impact I could have on such violent men I could never truly relate to. When the men arrived, I spoke for a few minutes, then took out my guitar and began singing the Prayer of St. Francis—"Lord, make me an instrument of your peace." When the meeting was finished, a tall, dangerous looking man approached me and asked if we could speak privately. I said yes, and he led me away from the group to a spot where we could speak alone. I felt my heart begin to race, wondering why he needed such privacy. When he finally stopped and turned around, I noticed tears running down his cheeks. "I've killed as many as five men in one day," he said, "and even though I don't know how to live the way you described, I want it." We looked at each other and something seemed to lock into place. As if on cue our arms opened, and we fell together into one of the most beautiful hugs I've ever experienced. I don't know how long we stood there, but I felt something change in him. Maybe the hug we shared created the opening he needed to make a new choice. I don't know, but I believe it's possible.

And I believe the possibilities of transforming ourselves and each other within the energy of a hug is real.

So why hold back? That's the real message of this book. Dr. Stone has done the world a great service by sharing his keen, clinical, pioneering perspective, and I truly believe that if you give a hug the time it deserves—then put it into practice—you will agree. It may be one of the simplest and most effective ways we have of breaking down boundaries and creating peace—and I mean that quite literally. My suggestion is to test it out for yourself. One of the biggest discoveries you'll make is that you will get as much out of the practice as the person you're offering the hug to. Isn't that the way it should be?

I could go on and on, but I really want you to get to Dr. Stone's masterpiece. He's the expert, not me. All I can say is that you wouldn't have been guided to this book unless you were ready for it, unless you realized that your hugs are powerful beyond belief. So keep turning the pages until you feel a light turn on inside you, then go give a few hugs and see what happens.

JAMES TWYMAN
New York Times bestselling author of *The Moses Code*
April 19, 2019

Author's Note

My intention in writing *Hug Therapy* is to offer information of a general nature to help you in your quest for emotional and spiritual well-being.

You are fully responsible for your own actions, which will be discussed in more detail throughout the book. By taking control of and full responsibility for your life, anything is possible. I cannot guarantee that everyone will receive your hugs in a positive way, and it is important that hugs are fully consensual. This is so important that an entire chapter is dedicated to its discussion. Enter and follow at your own risk, and know that seeing life through the lens of a hug can be pure magic.

Introduction

If I were there with you right now, I'd give you a great big hug. Nothing weird. Just a full-on, unconditional love hug. Allow me to introduce myself. I'm "the Hug Doctor" and the founder of "Hug Therapy." This book was written to be my hug to you. It's also a personal invitation from me to you… to embrace yourself, your life, and everyone around you in a whole new way.

Can you remember the last time someone gave you an all-encompassing hug like the one I just described? A boundless embrace with endless vibrations of gratitude and support that's so overpowering it squeezes every ounce of fear, worry, and negativity out of your spirit—leaving you with nothing but warmth, inner peace, and a feeling of connection?

Hug Therapy will make you feel like that, but it isn't just a "feel good" book. It's also a "do good" book that will help you live more in the moment and stay more tuned in with the things that matter to you most. You already know that the key to happiness isn't cramming more activities into your already busy life. It's about having the insight and vision to know what really matters to you, and being brave enough to take action in those areas.

This journey is a marathon, not a sprint, so it might not be easy or happen overnight, but it is simple, and anyone can do it.

Now you might be saying, "I'm not a hugger, and I'm not into all this touchy-feely shit." I hear you loud and clear, and appreciate you saying what you really think and feel (more about the value of expressing yourself directly later in the book). I strongly encourage you to keep reading. Not only because I'm selling this book for money, but seriously, because hugs come in many shapes and sizes, and hugging speaks to much more than a physical hug. Living in "the space of a hug" means being more accepting of yourself and everyone else; allowing you to be more appreciative of all life has to offer. You can do this without any physical hugging. And consider, that maybe, just maybe, you will feel very differently about physical hugging as the book unfolds.

Although giving and receiving physical hugs is part of the 21-Day "Hugging Journey™," Hug Therapy is so much more.

My 21-day hugging journeys have pushed me out of my comfort zone, deepened my connections, and super charged my passion for life. I couldn't be more excited for you to join me and experience the journey for yourself. I believe that as more and more people are inspired to go on hugging journeys, the energy and momentum of Hug Therapy will increase exponentially.

Hug Therapy

Hug Therapy can have a remarkable impact on any domain of our lives. Too often in life, we are on a path that has been worn so deeply that we feel sick, bored, or trapped. Even when we are excited about what we have achieved in one domain, we often struggle, wondering what else is out there. Sometimes in certain areas of life, we are firing on all cylinders, while in others, we feel lost. Some people have achieved financial success, and yet, feel trapped in an unhealthy relationship. Others may be in a beautiful relationship and no longer find meaning in other parts of life. The Hugging Journey allows you to look hard and assess what is working, what is not working, and then choose to take bold "hugging steps," allowing you to live more fully.

This Is How It Happened

What you are reading was conceived in an "ah-ha" moment. Books are often the result of much thinking and planning, sometimes for years, before the author sits down to write. This book had its beginnings in quite a different way. I had no intentions of writing a book, and certainly not one on this subject. This is how it happened.

...

My friend and I were on a tour of the breathtaking home, Fallingwater, a house designed by architect Frank Lloyd Wright in 1935, located in rural southwestern Pennsylvania, about an hour southeast of Pittsburgh. We ran into a fellow tourist (let's call him Sandy), whom I had seen in passing earlier that day. I was ready to move on when I had an uncharacteristic thought; it occurred to me that Sandy might need/want a hug. I didn't know him, I had never seen him until that morning, and I had no idea why that thought popped into my head. What's more, it wouldn't go away. *Why not*? I wondered. *I could use a hug; maybe he could, too.* The other side of my mind was having none of it. *He'll think you're crazy. He'll just walk away.* I settled the argument by walking up to Sandy

Hug Therapy

and saying, "Hi. My name is Stone. Would you like a hug?" Sandy hesitated for a moment, and then said, "Sure." So, we shared a solid hug as if we were old friends reconnecting after a long separation.

This was a powerful, restorative hug—our connection, however brief, was highly meaningful. I never asked Sandy how he felt about it; in fact, I never saw him again. I don't know whether I had sensed that he was silently asking for a hug or if one of us needed a hug. Whatever the reason, the result was transformative, at least for me.

The next hug was in Thermópolis, Wyoming, which I'm told is the largest natural hot springs in the world. While my daughter and I were in the ninety-nine-degree pool, I got into a conversation with a guy (let's call him Cody), who was also on vacation with his daughter. While the girls played together, Cody and I exchanged a little information. He told me he was planning to buy a place in Thermopolis as a second home; he lived in Colorado. After a while, we said our goodbyes and went our separate ways.

The next day, as I was going for a jog along the river, I saw him again. He had mentioned to me the day before that he was a huge fly fisherman. He was standing on the side of the river with his truck parked close by. Cody said his daughter was still asleep in the truck, and that they had stayed the night there, by the river.

As we chatted, we shared our divorce experiences. Mine was amicable; his was ugly. He and his ex-wife had fought over custody of their daughter for five years. It was a messy battle. At the end of our talk, I asked him if he would like a hug. I was pleased that he agreed. We had what I consider a significant hug for two people who recently met. It probably lasted for about fifteen or twenty seconds. I felt a deep platonic connection. I wished him well, and continued my run.

At that moment, I knew I was going to write *Hug Therapy*. I was as sure of it as I had ever been of anything in my life. I debated including this in the book and then, upon further reflection, I knew I wanted to be radically transparent with you. (More about radical transparency later.) What happened was as I jogged away, I heard a powerful voice state, "You will write a book about the power of hugging." This was jarring on many levels, and, in my state of shock, I simply replied, "Okay." From that moment on, this book has been my focus, and hugging, the center of my life. I now see everything through the lens of a hug. I will explain this new perspective throughout the book.

The fates, however, were not yet finished. My family and I were supposed to leave Thermopolis and spend a night in

Riverton, Wyoming, at the Wind River Casino. However, no one thought it made sense to do any extra driving, so we decided to stay another day. Back at the hot springs, I ran into Cody. We greeted each other as friends. Cody and I resumed our conversation, and, to my delight, he told me that following our hug the day before, he had walked around all morning with a smile he couldn't erase. I made a note to myself to put this in the book. By this point, it was like a one-two punch. The universe or something was telling me to write the book, and also confirming its impact. I became a HUGe believer in the power of hugging. This could make a difference in the world.

The next hug occurred in Mountain View, California, where I was sitting with my friend Earl at an outside patio restaurant, discussing the books each of us was writing. A couple sat nearby, engaged in a lively conversation. They seemed to be having a romantic date and were very much immersed in each other. During our dinner, I read a few pages of *Hug Therapy* to Earl to solicit his feedback and advice. As we left, the gentleman next to us, whose name was Stefano, apologized and said that he had something he felt compelled to share. He explained that he overheard much of our conversation and wanted me to know that I was on the right path. He told me a few times, "Go for it."

He also mentioned the Kabbalah (the ancient Jewish tradition of mystical interpretation of the Old Testament) and how much it meant to him. He thought it may be at the essence of what my book is about. Well, I was dumbfounded. For a stranger to approach me this boldly and supportively was jarringly positive. When I recovered from my surprise, I asked him if he would like a hug. He jumped out of his seat, as if he had been waiting for me to ask; he was clearly overjoyed. We shared a long, intense hug. Then Earl asked to hug Stefano's girlfriend. Next, our server, John, came out and got involved. Then, I had a warm embrace with Stefano's girlfriend. Earl took a picture of Stefano and me, and we exchanged contact information.

The upshot of this "hug fest" is that people you have just met may want to give you a hug. They may be quite conscious of wanting to do so, or the desire may be just below the surface. One can connect with a fellow human being at any moment. That connection is our common bond that says, "I want you to be in my life, if only for this instant." The hug may be a once-in-a-lifetime occurrence, as it was with Sandy, or it may be the beginning of a lifelong friendship. We don't really know. What matters is heartfelt contact with another person. In the best of all possible worlds, that person will feel moved to increase their hugging.

Of course, these are just a few of the meaningful hug interactions I've had, but they all told me I was going in the right direction. Since that time, I've expanded *Hug Therapy* to include exercises for embracing people you already know, yourself, and your life. The goal is to motivate people to make hugging a touchstone of what really matters in life.

Memoirist Bonnie Ware worked in palliative care for many years. In her book, *The Top Five Regrets of the Dying: A Life Transformed by the Dearly Departed*, she writes about patients' regrets as they look back on their lives. Most often mentioned is, "I wish I'd had the courage to live a life true to myself, not the life others expected of me."

Hug Therapy will help you live a life that is true to yourself, a life that is played full out, in which you left it all on the field, so to speak. This idea is captured brilliantly as *carpe diem* (seize the day), which many may recall from *Dead Poets Society*. In this movie, Robin Williams is a teacher who is passionately focused on helping his students go after what really matters to them. He reminds them, "We are food for worms, lads! Because we're only going to experience a limited number of springs, summers, and falls. One day, hard as it is to believe, each and every one of us is going to stop breathing, turn cold, and die!"

It is this same awareness that can allow us to look deeply and discover what really matters to us.

Part I

Hugging Essentials

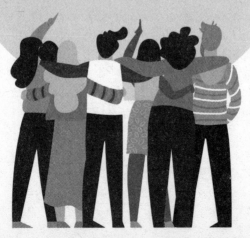

How to Use and Not Use This Book

Hug Therapy is divided into six parts.

Part I lays out the hugging essentials. It includes: a brief history of hugging, as well as the science behind *Hug Therapy*. Next, it provides an overview of the benefits of hugging, as conveyed in *The Hug Store*, a beautiful book about hugs, written from a child's perspective, to help better understand the important question "where do hugs come from?"

Then, the first section shifts into how common it is to feel stuck, and explores how a hug can be a tool to an increased awareness, moving us from feeling stuck, to being powerfully in action. It introduces the concepts of being fully grounded, appreciating ourselves, and truly embracing our value and completeness in this very moment.

Part II provides tools to utilize when planning your first 21-Day Hugging Journey. It introduces the concepts of *supercharged mindfulness* and *radical transparency* (truth in love). Next, Part II explores how *any* interaction between two people is either a hug or not a hug, and how identifying this can be helpful. It also introduces three different levels of hugging, including, "the space of a hug," the physical hug, and the virtual hug. Finally, and perhaps most importantly, this part includes the critical Action Steps to Starting Your 21-Day Hugging Journey (see page 91 if you want to jump ahead right now).

Part III explores what it means to Embrace Yourself—literally and figuratively—with sample exercises to guide you. It doesn't matter what you have or haven't done in the past. That is over. Loving yourself in this moment and taking care of you is at the core of *Hug Therapy*. Start to embrace that concept in *this* moment, accepting this and letting it wash over you. Too many of us hold onto anger, frustration, and resentment, allowing it to drag us down like a bag full of bricks. Let's work together to identify these heavy burdens, and then let go of them, so you can feel lighter and refreshed, with newfound energy and purpose. It helps to explore how you can surprise and delight yourself each day, and have increased awareness that you are the hero on this journey.

Part IV is about Embracing Life, with more exercises to help you appreciate and make the most of every moment. Together, we will come up with new ways to stimulate your creativity and set new goals. You will be encouraged to do all those things you've been thinking about doing, but haven't yet

Hug Therapy

taken on. It's action time! The way to make things happen is by putting a concrete structure in place.

Part V is about Embracing Others, with additional exercises to help you connect with the people in your life: family, friends, coworkers, neighbors, and even people you don't yet know. It's also about the critical importance of understanding the mutuality of a hug, and of being clear whether the huggee really wants a hug, with an important focus on "consensual hugging or not at all." You can't fully embrace yourself and life without embracing others(This doesn't necessarily mean physical hugging, it can also mean fully embracing them metaphorically, such as truly listening to them, hearing their story, and really seeing them). A huge part of hugging is about developing empathy, compassion, respect, and focusing on doing your best to truly understand this other person, so that you can be as supportive as they need in that moment.

Part VI is about bringing together all the different, rich forms of hugging that have been explored throughout *Hug Therapy*. It emphasizes deeply engaging in life through a 21-Day Hugging Journey that lights you up and inspires you. Whether you are already in action or about to begin, this section reminds us that the only day to really hug ourselves or anyone else is today. Hug yourself and those around you, and spread love and acceptance in the world.

Hug Therapy is for people of all walks of life and beliefs. That said, you might be interested to discover that the teachings you read here are inspired, in part, by the Kabbalah—the ancient Jewish wisdom that helps reveal how the universe and life work, which seeks to develop the following:

- A deep understanding of nature, the world, and who we are.

- Practical tools for developing a new perspective on the world around us.

- An awareness of the source of problems in our personal lives and in society.

Those are also the ambitious goals of *Hug Therapy*. As you read and work your way through each chapter, the goal is to come away with a powerful exploration of these areas. Each brief essay has three parts:

The author's thoughts and insights on the chapter's subject.

Why this matters (i.e. how you will benefit from incorporating this concept in your life).

Action steps and activities to apply what you've learned to your unique situation.

Allow *Hug Therapy* to guide you into a new hugging paradigm as your understanding of its principles and insights grow.

I hope you will come to think of it as a discovery source and launching pad. This is not a book to rush through and put back on the shelf. If you got a digital copy, it's perfect because you can have it with you whenever you want. This is a book to read in your quiet moments, to revisit often, and know it's there for you.

As you are reading *Hug Therapy* and engaging in the exercises, know that you are brave, wise, and unstoppable. This is not a pep talk. Whether you doubt any of it, even a little, or know it wholeheartedly, embark on this journey of discovery. It will open you up more and more to who you are and what you want. It will all happen through something so simple and straightforward that you may take it for granted: the hug.

The hug may be a large part of your day or a little piece of your week. It may be something you can't recall doing for a while or an activity you disdain—something only for those who are emotional or soft. You will be challenged, supported, and ultimately unleashed. It will all happen through your relationship with, and your understanding of the power of the hug.

Congratulations on embarking on a journey that, through your investment and labors, will reward you with powerful breakthroughs—both large and small—throughout your life.

Is it bold or naïve to suggest that *Hug Therapy* is potent enough to radically transform your life—and the planet? Perhaps. But I have a few things going for me. First, everyone understands the power of a hug. Second, most are capable of hugging. And, third, hugging is scientifically proven to have many positive effects. Of course, I'll tell you more about that in the coming chapters.

So, let's get started…and "hug it out!"

STONE

Hugging 101–Definitions Overview

Radical Transparency—Your word is extremely powerful when you act in accordance with your heart and stay true to yourself. Being aware of what you really think and feel in this moment, and expressing yourself will set you free.

Full Responsibility—You are masterful and fully accountable for your life. You can create anything you are fully committed to, and connect with others in doing so. This awareness is powerful. Seeing the world this way gives you access to action and how to create it through connection. This way of viewing the world offers you unique access to building and embracing a life that inspires you.

Regardless of your situation, you can change your life. Awareness of your present situation is your launching pad for moments, days, and years of unlimited possibility. It all begins with action today. This is about achieving the end result on the one hand, and—perhaps more importantly, and at least equally importantly—understanding who you know yourself to be in this moment, based on the action you take today. What if today was the last day you had to live? How would you want to know and love yourself? Not in any way bound to the balance in your bank account, retirement plan, or having the most toys, but in a more essential manner. How would you want to be with your loved ones and all the people around you? How would you embrace this moment and be fully engaged in life and the magic of you?

When you embrace each of these components, anything is possible. You will know with your entire being that you are a miracle, and that you can dance and play through life.

If you follow the recommendations here, you will begin to embrace yourself and the world, feel fully alive and present, and increase your potential to create deep connections wherever you go.

Brief History of Hugging

The official origin of where or when the act of hugging began is uncertain. It seems to be one of those instinctive behaviors humans share with primates to express emotional connection, love, consolation, and comfort. Wanting to be held in a tight embrace by another appears to be human instinct or primate instinct, and arguably, mammalian instinct. Human biology requires nurturing by our primary caretakers in order to thrive, because we can't care for ourselves as babies and children. A hug may often be used when words fail or seem insufficient.

When we stop to think about it, hugging likely goes back as far as human existence. Even when there was only one person in existence, that individual likely had an evolutionary focus on taking care of themself (a self-hug). Once there were two or more individuals, they likely bonded together to support each other, and for the propagation of the species.

Historically, offering a hug or a handshake demonstrated that neither individual had a weapon, and was a sign of good faith. It is also a gesture that can be seen in the art of many cultures throughout history and across the world.

The specific origins of the word "hug" are unclear, and two theories exist. The first suggests it to be of Scandinavian origin, and is often presumed to be connected to the Old Norse *hugga* (first used in 1560), which was understood to loosely mean "to comfort." The second, is that the word is related to the German word *hegen*, meaning to foster or cherish, and originally meant to enclose with a hedge.

TREE HUGGING

One distinct use of the word "hug" is tied to "tree hugging," which was first identified in India in the 1700s. The legend goes that when the maharajah wanted to build a new palace, he planned to build it on the land of the Bishnoi people, to whom trees are sacred. The Bishnoi people worship nature, and thus, the killing of anything in nature, including trees, is forbidden. A female villager noticed men about to cut down the precious Kherjri trees, and positioned herself between the men and the trees, wrapping herself tightly around the tree, legend says, hugging it with all her might. She is said to have offered her head if it would save one tree, and the maharajah's loggers chopped her head off with an axe.

The story goes that three other girls, and eventually hundreds of Bishnoi villagers, responded in the same way, joining the protest. Legend has it that 353 people had been murdered before the maharajah ordered a decree protecting the land from future harm. To this day, logging and hunting in Bishnoi villages is still prohibited.

Through the years, tree-hugging has continued to be a means of peaceful resistance to prevent the lumber industry from destroying native forests. It has become a more common way for environmentalists to protest, as well as become a part of green spiritualist practice.

AMMA

One distinct and extremely influential and powerful hugger is Amma. She was born into a low caste family in the fishing village of Parayakadavu in the district of Kerala in India on September 27, 1953. Her parents remarked that she was born into the world smiling, and not crying. She grew up very different from other children in that she was very spiritual, and it is said that even at age five, she was spending much of her time praying. When she was nine, her parents sent her off to school, and she was given the worst jobs to do, which she did gladly. As she grew older, her mystical experiences intensified, and she began to gain followers attracted to her spirituality. Her devotees often said she took on the form of Sri Krishna, and many miraculous healings have been attributed to her.

Amma is uneducated in the traditional sense, but she teaches her followers about the ancient traditions of Yoga and Vedanta. Her main teaching has been to reject the false sense of ego, and focus on the divine, true nature of man. During the past thirty-five years, her main focus has been to travel the world and offer unconditional love to people from all walks of life. It is estimated that Amma has hugged over *thirty-three million people worldwide*. On some days, she may have hugged up to fifty thousand people in a day, working for up to twenty hours.

She does not try to convert people to her religion, and says that her "sole mission is to love and serve one and all." Some people claim to feel vibrations when they hug her. They have come to see that her hugs are not just physical, but are spiritually powerful, and her touch is a blessing. Because she hugs for hours, her stamina and presence seem almost otherworldly. It is that endurance that gives her the magnetism people call saintly.

NATIONAL HUGGING DAY

Kevin Zaborney is credited with the creation of National Hugging Day in 1986. It is also known as National Hug Day, International Hug Day, and Global Hug Day. This immensely important observance occurs annually on January 21 and was first celebrated in Michigan. It is now celebrated all over the world. Zaborney explained that the idea of National Hugging Day was to encourage everyone to hug family and friends more often. He chose the time of year for National Hugging Day because it is the emotionally low period following Christmas/New Years and before Valentine's Day. The benefits of hugging are extensive, and in part, can reduce blood pressure, increase self-esteem, and improve both physical and mental health.

Zaborney cautions people to ask first if uncertain of the response, out of respect for personal boundaries. Zaborney has traveled all over the world promoting National Hugging Day. He is a founding member of the National Hugging Alliance, which worked with the Guinness World Records to set the benchmark for a world record of the Most Nationalities in a Group Hug. That effort successfully brought together more than forty-three different nationalities in the world's first 21-Second Hug on January 21, 2018.

FREE HUG MOVEMENT

In 1999, Bernard and Delia Carey started an extraordinary social movement by washing people's feet in New York City. They placed a sandwich board sign out on the street, and waited for people to come in, no donations, and no fuss.

People started getting curious and stopping into the little storefront on East 10th Street. Before long, the Careys were offering hugs, bandages, and money. The biggest letters outside the store were the ones that read "Free Hugs."

What began as a storefront whim became an artistic experience. Customers referred to it as "performance," but the Careys wanted to do something bigger and more impactful. They delved into the idea of "relational aesthetics," traced back to the 1960s interdisciplinary community, Fluxus, which included performances by artists like Yoko Ono.

They began taking pictures and videotaping their experiences, and, before long, their "Free Hugs" became a national news story. They were asked to be in the Whitney Biennial Art Show in New York City, where they gave out hugs and were interviewed on the morning news program *Good Morning America*. The Biennial happened in 2002, in the wake of 9/11, and the Careys' exhibit served as a public source of comfort for still grieving Americans. Most importantly, they were able to get the public to think of hugs as a service, something that people could give and receive much more from in return.

In May 2004, a man named Jonathan Littman began giving out hugs in Washington Square Park in New York City every Sunday, under a sign labeled "Free Hugs." He also traveled to

Germany and did the same. He wanted to utilize and share his generosity with the people around him.

One month later, in June 2004, it was reported that Juan Mann gave out hugs for the first time in Sydney, Australia in exactly the same way Littman had done. But Juan included a viral video as well. The band Sick Puppies created a music video out of his travels that became an instant internet success. Juan Mann began giving out hugs, because he wanted to be hugged. Millions of people have watched his video, and although Mann retired from the Free Hug movement in 2009, the video continues to inspire.

Ken Nwadike Jr. is a documentary filmmaker and peace activist known as the "Free Hug Guy." He attended the 2014 Boston Marathon to spread love and encourage runners with free hugs. He explained, "while viewing the devastation of the 2013 bombing of the Boston Marathon, I was determined to be a participant in the next race. I failed to qualify by just twenty-three seconds, so I decided to attend the event in a different way." He provided free hugs for runners in the marathon, and this simple act of encouragement resulted in national headlines. The hugs resulted in smiles and gave runners an extra boost of energy. He has invigorated the free hugs movement, and explains that the mission of the *Free Hugs Project* is to continue the work of Dr. Martin Luther King

Jr., "to spread love, inspire change, and raise awareness of social issues."

The Science Behind Hug Therapy: A Word with Dr. Kipp

To explain oxytocin from a medical standpoint, I asked my friend and colleague Dr. Kipp to share his expertise. Dr. Kipp is an interventional radiologist and former family practitioner. He is triple board certified, and has an extensive formal education, including medical training with two residencies and a fellowship covering a span of nine years of post-graduate education. Dr. Kipp speaks all over the country about issues ranging from the human-animal bond to the Affordable Care Act, and the sanctity of the patient-doctor bond. He is also the host of the radio talk show called *Doctor's Orders*.

Have you ever watched a mother with her newborn baby? It doesn't matter whether you're participating in the birth of a child or of an animal in nature. The moment the child is born, the natural bond between mother and newborn forms, permanent, durable, and everlasting. Mothers love to cuddle with their newborns. They love the touch of their infants upon their skin. They even describe the distinct smell of their babies.

Animal studies have shown similar results. Mother horses know their own foal, even in a crowded pen of newborn colts. Mother mice are able to identify their pups in a crowded cage, and if the pup is separated from the mother for a short period of time, upon return, the mother showers her baby with maternal affection by licking its fur.

Have you ever wondered why? Childbirth has been described as the greatest possible pain any human will ever experience. When people have any other pain in their lives, they tend to avoid and run from the negative stimulus as fast as their legs can carry them. What is it, then, that makes a mother immediately forget the pain and suffering (sometimes as long as eighteen to twenty hours of pain)? And I mean immediately. It must be something powerful.

It is. Science has analyzed, examined, and studied this phenomenon for years, and has discovered some amazing things. Although an entire neurological system is working in unison before, during, and after the delivery, the one specific chemical that appears to have the most profound effect is oxytocin.

Oxytocin is a neuropeptide, which simply means it is a natural chemical, a hormone, produced by the hypothalamus in the brain. All scientific data points to oxytocin as the number-one explanation for a mother immediately forgetting that pain. If this hormone can have such an extraordinary effect during childbirth, what effect will it have on our everyday lives?

A well-known study at the University of North Carolina in Chapel Hill highlighted just how powerful oxytocin can be.[1]

The research includes studying oxytocin release in married couples and cohabiting adults. For ten minutes, the scientists in the lab ask the couple to spend time holding hands, hugging each other, and reminiscing about pleasurable events in their life, like how they met and how they fell in love. The couples then had their blood drawn for evaluation of oxytocin levels, and filled out a questionnaire. The results were telling—those couples who had higher oxytocin levels had better relationships. Science has begun to realize the valuable benefits of oxytocin. More study is necessary to fully understand the effects, and these studies are ongoing.

The dopamine-response system in the brain, under the influence of oxytocin, controls our ability to perceive pleasure. These neuropeptides, oxytocin and dopamine, have become known as endorphins, or pleasure chemicals. Here are some things we do know about oxytocin and hugs: When we

---

1 Light, Kathleen C., Karen M. Grewen, and Janet A. Amico. "More frequent partner hugs and higher oxytocin levels are linked to lower blood pressure and heart rate in premenopausal women." University of North Carolina at Chapel Hill. 2005. https://uncch. pure.elsevier.com/en/publications/more-frequent-partner-hugs-and-higher-oxytocin-levels-are-linked-.

embrace someone, oxytocin is released, and this makes us feel warm and fuzzy. This promotes feelings of devotion, trust, and bonding. The touch also enables the participants to develop a stronger sense of acceptance, and decreases loneliness, isolation, and depression. But it's more than that—the hug leads to the lowering of one's blood pressure. This appears to be directly related to improvement, or a decrease, in cortisol, the stress hormone. The same oxytocin effect can happen when you hug or interact with a pet. Besides being at the root of the human-human bond, oxytocin is also instrumental in the positive changes observed in the human-animal bond.

The UNC study results tell us some interesting things about human contact, specifically hugs. When a person experiences the inviting touch of another person, a burst of chemicals fills the brain with a wave of warmth. Oxytocin is released, and the pleasure receptors are bathed in pleasure chemicals.

What does this mean for the science behind the hug? Everything. It brings our emotional self in line with our physical self. Science provides the validation that something pleasing has occurred. And it's even more profound than that, although there is some controversy on whether how the duration of the hug determines how much oxytocin is released, with some scientists claiming a twenty-second hug is needed for any oxytocin release. Recent studies raise the possibility that oxytocin release starts seconds before humans' exchange contact. Just thinking about a hug may have a similar, if not identical, effect as the actual thing.

Remember the phrase "an apple a day keeps the doctor away?" Medical professionals have analyzed this statement from various angles. What if we changed it to "a hug a day"? Interestingly, a new study at Carnegie Mellon University, involving 404 healthy adults, studied the effect of a hug on their overall susceptibility to developing the common cold after being exposed to the rhinovirus.[2]

People who perceived greater social support from hugging showed a 32 percent decreased risk in developing the common cold. And even those who developed a cold experienced less pronounced symptoms, if they perceived a positive benefit from hugging, and received more frequent hugs. It appears that hugging protects people who are under stress from the increased risks for colds usually associated with stress. Hugging is a marker of intimacy, and helps generate the feeling that others are there to help in the face of adversity. Psychologists have described hugging as follows: hugs surround the recipient with a "force field," or an

---

2   Rea, Shilo. "Hugs Help Protect Against Stress and Infection, Say Carnegie Mellon Researchers." Carnegie Mellon University. December 17, 2014. https://www.cmu.edu/news/stories/archives/2014/december/december17_hugsprotect.html.

invisible armor that gives the person a psychological feeling of safety and security.[3] [4]

What's more telling is what is exactly happening at the physiological level. When the person receives the hug, touch, or human contact, this stimulates pressure receptors under your skin in a way that leads to a cascade of events, including an increase in vagal activity. Specifically, stimulation of the vagus nerve triggers the hypothalamus to release oxytocin. The increase in oxytocin levels in the bloodstream creates a domino effect in which the adrenal glands inhibit or decrease the amount of cortisol and norepinephrine in the bloodstream. These effects place you in a relaxed, contented, and secure state. Another related study from the University of North Carolina School of Medicine in Chapel Hill studied postpartum mothers. They found that higher oxytocin levels were associated with lower cardiovascular and sympathetic-nervous reactivity to stress.[5]

---

3   Polard, Andrea F., PsyD. "4 Benefits of Hugs, for Mind and Body." *Psychology Today.* June 8, 2014. https://www.psychologytoday.com/blog/unified-theory-happiness/201406/4-benefits-hugs-mind-and-body.

4   Jakubiak, Brittany K., and Brooke C. Feeney. "Affectionate Touch to Promote Relational, Psychological, and Physical Well-Being in Adulthood." Personality and Social Psychology Review. March 24, 2016. http://journals.sagepub.com/doi/abs/10.1177/1088868316650307.

5   Grewen, Karen M., and Kathleen C. Light. "Plasma oxytocin is related to lower cardiovascular and sympathetic reactivity to stress." ISI Articles. 2011. http://isiarticles.com/bundles/Article/pre/pdf/39086.pdf.

Indeed, a hug a day—especially a twenty-one-second hug—may very well keep the doctor away.[6]

What could this mean for long-term treatment of stroke victims during their physical rehabilitation, situational or even chronically depressed patients and their daily medical regimen? Could frequent hugs, or so many quality hugs a day, be prescribed as part of their medical therapy? Why not include a prescription that states, "Three twenty-one-second hugs a day, every day"? And for stressful conditions, add a fourth thirty-second hug when needed. Why not? There's enough physical evidence to suggest hugs provide the recipient with measurable and reproducible benefits.

The scientific community hopes that anxiety patients may be helped more quickly with the aid of oxytocin. Oxytocin would have a positive effect on the patient's perception of fear. It would aid in bonding between therapist and subject, suggesting a heightened increase in success of treatment. Oxytocin could become an alternative to standard anxiolytics like lorazepam or diazepam, but with a much more natural approach, and less risk of side effects. More clinical studies are needed, but early results suggest there is reason for much optimism. Oxytocin may change how we look at and treat

6   Colino, Stacey. "The Health Benefits of Hugging." U.S. News & World Report. February 03, 2016. http://health.usnews.com/health-news/health-wellness/articles/2016-02-03/the-health-benefits-of-hugging.

anxiety in the future. The possibilities are virtually endless, or at least that's how it seems now.

We see anecdotal examples every day. "When I come home, my daughter will run to the door and give me a big hug, and every stress that happened that day just melts away." I doubt this father knew much about science, or that he understands the oxytocin effect behind this display of love and affection, but his statement speaks to the depth of his grasp of the hidden benefits behind his daughter's hug. If hugs can have this level of influence on our daily lives, shouldn't we incorporate human contact into our daily activities? I suspect we would all be much better for it as individuals, as families, and as fellow citizens of the world. If someone important has passed on from this world, what would you give to have the chance to hug them once more? Don't be afraid to touch your loved ones—your health and well-being may depend on it.

The Benefits of Hugging from *The Hug Store*

1. Reduces stress, worry, and anxiety

2. Increases calmness

3. Reduces production of cortisol (the stress hormone)

4. Enhances bonding differently than language alone

5. Lowers levels of emotional and physical pain

6. Increases compassion and understanding

7. Relieves depression

8. Elevates mood

9. Boosts and enhances the immune system

10. Relaxes muscles in the body

11. Lowers blood pressure and improves heart health

12. Balances the nervous system

13. Reduces feelings of hostility and anger

14. Helps with nonverbal communication

15. Boosts self-esteem

The previous page is an excerpt from a children's book that I think offers a profound lesson. If you are looking for a great children's book, I suggest you read *The Hug Store* from Veronica Lane Books, written by father/daughter team Shana and Rick Morrison. It is based on a true story in which Shana (a five-year-old kindergartner) tells her grandfather that she "is all out of hugs" and needs "to go to the hug store to get more."

Feeling Stuck

Sadly, people often feel a nagging sense of dissatisfaction with their lives. Things are not turning out as they had hoped. They had plans that never materialized, goals and expectations they didn't meet, or dreams they never pursued. Their lives are full of shoulds: *I should be more successful. I should have gone back to school. I should be in better shape. My marriage should be happier.*

Perhaps you have thought, *I'm an unpaid chauffeur, driving my kids to lessons and practices and play dates. I resent being in this position, but I'm stuck.* You're comparing yourself to all the other parents and wondering about their levels of contentment as they drive kids to piano lessons or dancing lessons and hockey practices. *Is this the way my life should be?*

Or, maybe you are frustrated with your professional life. You may be thinking, *I'm in a job that's going nowhere. Half the time I'm bored, and the other half I'm frenzied and about to burn out. I don't like what I'm doing—it's a bad fit for my skills—but I'm stuck. Jobs are not that easy to find, and I should be happy I even have one. I have to support my family even if I don't love what I'm doing.*

Shoulds can lead you to a pity party: *My marriage should have worked out. I should be in better shape. I should be making more money. I should be married. I should go back to school, because I'm not getting anywhere. I should have gone for another degree or pursued a career in a different field.*

Does this sound familiar? Are there areas of your life that aren't working? If you feel overwhelmed, dissatisfied, or just plain stuck, you are not alone.

WHY THIS MATTERS

You are not stuck. By becoming aware of how you feel about your life, you have taken the first step on a life-changing journey. *Hug Therapy* is your guidebook.

ACTION

In all of life, and as you read the upcoming chapters, it is critical to identify what is and isn't the truth. As humans, we are prone to getting caught up in the drama of our lives. You must learn to separate what's actually true from your version of the truth. This must be done with razor precision. The challenge is that we get so caught up in our version of reality that we see it as the truth, even though an objective outsider will clearly see the distinction. Let *Hug Therapy* help you identify this difference. The value in it is immeasurable.

Begin to rely very heavily on these two questions: *Did that really happen?* and *Am I completely certain that actually happened?* For example, your best friend unexpectedly misses your birthday party. Many of us in a situation such as this have thoughts, like: *They don't really care about me. Are they really my best friend if they aren't willing to go out of their way to attend my birthday? A best friend shouldn't behave like this.* In this instance, the reality is that they did not physically attend the party. The rest is conjecture, and yet we often treat "the rest" as if it is fact. As a result, we often create a world of suffering, and become trapped in it. Open yourself to looking deeply at assumptions that you have made about the people in your life. Are you doing this to some of the people with whom you are or have been close? Getting lost in these inaccurate versions of reality is not only hurting ourselves and negatively impacting our quality of life, it is pulling ourselves away from the people in our world.

> "Each day of human life contains joy and anger, pain and pleasure, darkness and light, growth and decay. Each moment is etched with nature's grand design—do not try to deny or oppose the cosmic order of things."
>
> **—Morihei Ueshiba**

Dear Reader,

Consider that you are part of nature, perfect the way you are. In today's world, it's hard to accept that you are whole the way you are. We are constantly being fed advertising that says we need to change. This is nonsense, because you are as perfect as any part of nature.

Deeply connect with the moment you're in, regardless of where you are or who you are with.

Think of this book as your coach, and the message below as foundational. You will be encouraged to explore and embrace places and things you thought were too much or too hard. You can do this. Let the words below remind you of your power and completeness. Let them ground you in your place as a loving being who is capable of anything you conceive and pursue.

It was written with love, and you are encouraged to fully embrace it. Preferably read it aloud or listen to it online as you prepare for the journey ahead.

When All is Said and Done (a Message and Wake-Up Call)

Below is an example of one moment in life in which I was fully present. Look at it and use it as a tool to slow down and connect with yourself in any moment of your life that you choose.

We have this moment and only this moment.

You've likely heard the above statement many times. The challenge and the profound reality are to really "get" this in as many waking moments as possible.

It's 6:36 a.m. on a Thursday morning, and I'm looking out the bedroom window into a forest. In the foreground is a beautiful, gnarled tree with many bends and expressions. Alone, it stands proudly, and yet, it is not alone. It is surrounded by others, and the depth and the richness of the rest of the forest is captivating.

There are a few suggestions of green pushing through with new spring growth, but mostly there are shades of brown. The light is coming softly through the canopy of the forest and highlighting the various trees; some thicker, some thinner. And yet, the whole picture is woven together in a magical way. It's perfect. I can hear the birds chirping lightly in the background, and occasionally, the sound of a car passing by.

I want you to know that wherever you are in this moment, it's perfect, and it really works.

You can slow down, really notice your surroundings, and be with them. The acceptance of this morning, or whatever time of day it is right now as you're reading this, wherever you are, is the foundation for moving anywhere.

Accept that you are perfect, whole, and complete—not as an intellectual thing, not like "Yeah, I know, Stone." Instead, accept yourself as an embodiment of something in nature. You are perfect in the same way that each one of the hundreds of trees I see out my window is perfect.

Some are thinner; some are in bands together; some are wavy, and bumping into others. The taller ones that have the blue sky blasting out in the background, and the shorter ones that are waiting to grow; each branch, each piece of bark, each leaf—that is you and me, perfect.

Let this wash over you.

Any time you feel overwhelmed or lost, come back to this, and get in touch with how you are—as perfect as any stone; as whole and complete as a diamond, an amethyst, a ruby, or a boulder.

You have everything, and thus, need nothing. You may want things, and you may definitively create things, but know that you already have it all. Consider that from this foundation, you are already being the magic of who you really are.

This is not a pep talk. This is reality. You are perfect, whole, and complete. This is simply the reality, and you are either in touch with this reality or not.

Return to this meditation anytime you need or want to be reminded of your connection to the whole and to the magic of you. The meditation is twofold. On the one hand, it is a tool that can be used for grounding. On the other, its objective is to get you to fully invest yourself in any moment when you feel lost and disconnected—regardless of where you are. Wherever you are, be present, and utilize all your senses to slow down and identify that you are an interwoven piece of the fabric of the world. Wherever you are, recognize your connection to humanity, and the depth of this connection. Use it to regain your balance, and have a clearer, enhanced awareness of who you really are.

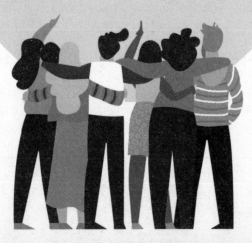

Part II

How to Hug

The following tools will help you powerfully engage in *Hug Therapy* and your 21-Day Hugging Journey.

Supercharged Mindfulness

Better understanding human survival instincts is the pathway to freedom. It gives us access to something other than our automatic response. Any time we feel threatened on any level, we do one of three things: fight, flee, or freeze. We either prepare to defend ourselves, try to escape, or shut down like a steel trap. This is our biology and the reality of our operating system. We don't have conscious control over our reaction to a threat. And face it—times have changed since the development of our operating system. I don't see any saber-toothed tigers around. We often have an *overly active* survival mechanism.

What if we had control over this mechanism? What if we lived in a world in which we knew we were safe? What would that world be like?

The key to a conscious life is awareness, moment to moment, which can be extremely difficult to maintain. We are like fish swimming in water. We don't generally notice we are focused on the past or the future, just as the fish doesn't notice the water. When it's all you know; of course, it becomes invisible.

We need a method to determine whether we are present in any given moment. This can be any mindfulness or meditation tool that you find effective. Do you have one that works for you? How often and effectively are you using it? Supercharged mindfulness is just this kind of tool.

Have you ever driven to the office or some other familiar destination and, when you arrived, had no memory of the trip? You've taken the same route hundreds of times; your car seems to go there without any help from you. You were on autopilot with your mind otherwise engaged. You are not alone. Most of us sleepwalk through life. We do things out of habit without even thinking. It's as if we are two people: one performing a task, and the other fixated on something else entirely.

The opposite of autopilot is mindfulness—total awareness of what you are doing and feeling, and what is going on around you at this moment. Mindfulness is something we crave to understand, with much research underway about its value and curative effects. In the early seventies, Ram Dass (formerly known as Richard Alpert), introduced the concept in his bestselling book *Be Here Now*. Mindfulness meditation is one of the steps in Buddhism's eightfold path. Psychologists are using it to help returning veterans with PTSD, and others who suffer from depression and anxiety. The point of mindfulness, according to Jon Kabat-Zinn, an author and expert on the subject, is to show up for more of the moments in our lives, instead of completely missing many of them.

Beyond mindfulness is a state called supercharged mindfulness, an awareness of the inner conflict between your automatic response and your intentional response. There are two ways to respond to any situation: automatically and intentionally. Here is an example of an automatic response: you notice someone, and you feel attracted to them. You walk over in an attempt to make a connection. But your automatic response kicks in. Your doubts surface. Fear takes over. *This is not a good idea*, you tell yourself. They don't know you, and probably wouldn't want to talk to you. They could even be offended if you say hello. So, you walk away without saying a word. Your automatic, self-protective impulse was to avoid risk and rejection. Though it may sound dramatic, you were in survival mode, an overly active one.

But, let's say that when you notice someone to whom you are attracted, you suspend your automatic warning system. You decide to go over and start a conversation. You have no idea how they might respond. But whether they say, "Hi, what's your name?" or "Excuse me. I don't talk to strangers," you feel very much alive. You made something happen that would not have happened if you had walked away. You created something. You know yourself to be someone who, although afraid, is also powerful, and acts on what matters. It's not that your automatic voices disappear. They continue to sound alarms; that's their job. They are making sure you survive, but you are discovering that you can ignore them, and not only survive, but thrive. You can still hear them, but you don't let them run the show. You can shut them down, and move toward what really matters to you. So, you introduce yourself to that intriguing other, and, as you talk to them, you focus more on them and less on your automatic voices. Now, you are creating rich possibilities for a potential new friend, business partner, or romantic interest. Regardless, in that moment, you know yourself to be someone who is living life, and really connecting with others and the world, all within the space of a hug.

What makes supercharged mindfulness distinct and immeasurably valuable?

Even when you think you are conscious of your actions and have done something on purpose, contemplate the possibility that your action had nothing to do with you. How can that be? The human condition is so profoundly trapped on autopilot, that we often don't notice when we are there. We are like that fish in the water; we don't realize what water is. The movie *The Matrix* portrays this false reality brilliantly; if you like the sci-fi genre, check it out. It depicts a dystopian future in which the reality that humans believe they exist in is actually not real, but created by sentient machines to use humans as an energy source.

Here is another example: if someone gives you a compliment, your response, no matter what it is, is an automatic thought over which you have no control. It is not the real you. In other words, you don't have to be conscious or aware to respond to the compliment. In fact, you don't have any control over your response. It is completely involuntary. There is nothing you can do about it, almost as though you are preprogrammed, and in a sense, you are.

Your mind is like a computer that has been recording everything that has happened in your life—every experience, every word, every emotion—and what it means in terms of your survival. Your mental computer has only one purpose: to keep you safe. To override this process, you must be aware of it. When you are on autopilot, you are unaware.

Let's go back to the compliment you received. Someone said something nice to you. You reacted automatically. A split second later, you became aware it was an automatic thought. Once you're aware that you're in the automatic mode, you have the power to break free, and then you can say or do anything. When this awareness occurs, you are completely alive. At that moment, anything is possible.

WHY THIS MATTERS

When you are aware of living on autopilot, that awareness gives you a freedom to dance and play in life. Yes, you already had an automatic response, but now that you are aware, you can create something new out of thin air that is totally representative of who you are and what really matters to you. Much of what you do or say to your boss, your partner, and your children isn't planned, thought out, or intentional; it's like a reflex. Once you notice the reflex, then you can actually share *you*—radically transparently.

Imagine you're with your two-year-old son, and he is acting like a two-year-old, and your buttons are getting pushed. You have lost your patience and let him know it. This has happened automatically, and you are instantly sorry that you scolded him. When you notice that you have raised your voice, you can immediately create a better scenario. For example, you might burst into a silly song in which you apologize on his level. "Daddy was so loud right now, like a silly cow somehow—moo, moo, moo—and you have so much energy, it's magical to me, and sometimes I get all wiggly." Silly, certainly, and how do you think that kiddo will be feeling about a parent who is smiling and playing? This is another example of the space of a hug. Or you might say, "I know I sounded angry, and I'm sorry. I love you, and I'm working hard to not do that again." A third possibility is to grab some crayons and quietly draw a picture together. None of these options is necessarily the right one for you. The beauty of supercharged mindfulness is that it allows you to create something new, something fun that works better in the moment. You won't change the behavior that has already happened, and, in *this* moment, you can be powerful, free, healing, loving, and fun. The alternative that we get stuck in way too frequently is victim mode. What good will it do to beat yourself up for having yelled at the child? What impact does getting caught in a pity party have in the moment of your engagement and awareness with the people you love? Start to look closely at how this is an anti-hug for each of us.

There are two ways to know whether you are experiencing supercharged mindfulness. One is that you will feel *alive*— animated, alert. It doesn't matter what you're doing; what matters is that you are completely aware and awake while you're doing it. This doesn't necessarily mean you are going to feel good. It might be like how alive you feel before going onstage to give a speech to a thousand people. I'm going to assert that although it may feel anxiety-provoking, that feeling, and knowing in the moment that you are alive, is a good thing. Step out into the world around you and hug it!

The second way is to change something that would not happen if you didn't take the initiative to make it happen. If the change you bring about could have occurred on its own, without you doing anything, then it is not supercharged mindfulness. This change must be something you choose to create, not something in which you are not involved. You may have read that last sentence and thought, "I don't get this. What the heck is he talking about?" For example, if your best friend is going to take you to a favorite dinner spot for your birthday—likely, you can see how the whole evening will play out in your mind's eye. You have likely been out together hundreds of times, and can probably imagine the place, the decor, the food, and the way you will be with your friend. Hypothetically, he will discuss his frustration with his mom, and you, your excitement about your new job, and what it's like to be a year older. To be clear, I'm not necessarily saying this is problematic. It could be a lovely evening. However, if it's happening automatically without your active participation, you aren't creating it. Perhaps you make a rule about not talking about his mom or your job—that would be creating. I'm not saying that's the right option, just one example. Let's say you have made a new friend, and you invite this third person to join you, and meet your old friend. That would be creating. Let's say that you sing "Happy Birthday" in Spanish to yourself while dancing around the restaurant and introducing yourself to strangers. That would be creating. Anything that has you stepping outside of your comfort zone—dancing, playing, and really connecting with the power of each moment—is creating.

This is a tough concept to understand, let alone execute. It takes a lot of tuning into your thoughts and realizing when they are instinctual, rather than intentional. The more often you can do this, the more aware you will become. Like any other skill, this takes practice. It's also helpful to accept and be aware that we spend much of life sleepwalking.

If you doubt whether your engagement in any activity is automatic or created, consider those doubts as a means to be certain that it's automatic. When you are fully alive and creating in the moment, you will know it beyond a shadow of a doubt.

How can we be alive? What tools discussed here could transform today from one in which we are mindlessly surviving to one in which we are passionately thriving? The answer lies in being superchargedly mindful, radically transparent with yourself and others, and aware that this moment might never pass our way again.

For example, as you wake up, you ask yourself if you want to exercise today—does it serve you in this moment? You look at your automatic reaction to that question, and realize you don't have to settle for what is there at first. You might choose to, but you don't have to. You are choosing how best to spend your moments, which allows you to give a self-hug. Some mornings it will be yes, and other mornings a no, and you note how that feels. The rest of the morning, you continue to stay attuned and pull yourself back when you get caught up in the past or future. You smell the coffee and notice the taste. You connect with your kids or friends and share your love and gratitude with them. Pay attention throughout your day, note how you feel, accept reality, and let go of the rest. Be patient with yourself as you notice you have lost minutes thinking about what needs to happen tomorrow or what you wished you did yesterday. The goal here is to notice the sweetness and poignancy in each moment, and when possible notice it could be your last moment.

In the play *Our Town* by Thorton Wilder, the main character, Emily, who is deceased, says:

"Let's really look at one another! …It goes so fast. We don't have time to look at one another. I didn't realize. So all that was going on and we never noticed…Wait! One more look. Goodbye. Goodbye, world…Goodbye to clocks ticking…and Mama's sunflowers. And food and coffee. And new ironed dresses and hot baths…and sleeping and waking up. Oh earth, you are too wonderful for anybody to realize you. Do any human beings ever realize life while they live it—every, every minute?"

Life can be hectic and stressful and crazy. You have the power to profoundly create. Be in *this* moment. Look for opportunities to give a 21-second hug. This includes longer physical hugs, but also other powerful ways of connecting that don't involve physical touch, the metaphorical 21-second hugs. Utilize radical transparency to be authentically alive and simultaneously engaged and thus lost in the moment.

ACTION

Think about tomorrow, and realize how many of the things you do every day that are automatic. Not only that, you can't remember most of them. Spontaneity is something you can create and play with when you are using supercharged mindfulness. This makes all the difference between indifference and passion. The experience of engagement and connection isn't dependent on who you are with or what you are doing—it's your connection between yourself and the world. Be inspired in *this* moment. Know yourself to be someone who is living in the space of a hug and being playful, alive, and embracing life—the good, the bad, and the ugly.

Hug/Not Hug

Any interaction between two people is either a hug or not a hug. Any interaction. It may be as simple as holding the door open for another person. What makes it a hug is the way in which you do it. If you genuinely smile at the other person, that's a hug; if you seem indifferent or rushed, not a hug. This is a very subtle and important concept. It often has less to do with action than with attitude. It has everything to do with awareness and how you view and experience yourself in that moment.

If you open the door grudgingly, or feel annoyed at how quickly or slowly the person walks through it—not a hug. If the focus is on how the other person *should* be behaving, then the moment is lost, and you are caught up in your own thoughts—not a hug. You have chosen to do something positive, and now you are feeling sorry for yourself. It all comes down to the way you are experiencing yourself. If holding the door open is truly a hug, you will feel the positive energy of being kind. This means moving away from self-focus, analysis, and judgment, and allowing yourself to feel the spark of connection and life. If you allow yourself to be in the "space of a hug," this feeling occurs, regardless of the other person's response. If they beam back at you and say thanks, this may intensify the spark. No matter their reaction to your behavior, you can experience the connection of being in the space of a hug, and know yourself as a kind and generous person.

Seeing the world through the lens of hugging allows us to slow down and witness our own behavior. Any behavior we engage in can either open ourselves up, which is a hug, or shut ourselves down—not a hug. Understanding this concept, and how to view life through the lens of a hug will open the door to possibility.

WHY THIS MATTERS

Viewing the world through the lens of hugging allows you to live a life in which you don't let self-pity take over your days, weeks, or months. Keep in mind, it is normal to feel sorry for yourself, but if it happens regularly, you need to become aware of it, and cancel the pity party.

The human condition, for better or worse, is to blame others for almost everything that goes wrong. Your coach (this book) is designed to give you concrete tools to notice when you are stuck in your head and get you back into life. In any moment, you can ask yourself, *Was that a hug?* Don't judge or beat yourself up about the answer to that question. Just pay close attention to what's a hug and what's not. Being fully conscious of your feelings will create a deeper level of connection with the people you love, as well as with yourself. It will increase your patience, peace of mind, and sense of your place in the world.

ACTION

It's time to make an investment in changing your behavior. Without action, understanding how to view your interactions with others through the lens of a hug on a conceptual level alone is of limited value.

To make it count, list three people with whom you struggle. Pay close attention to how you ordinarily deal with those people, and how it would change if you viewed them through the lens of a hug. There are two parts to this exercise: First, be aware how it feels to make your attitude and behavior more loving. Second, notice what happens to these relationships when you view them in a new way and change your behavior.

What if nothing happens? What if the relationships continue to be difficult? Have you failed? Not at all. Whether these relationships stay the same or improve isn't the primary focus. What matters is your attitude, your behavior, and your awareness of both. Essentially, you have created a hug by changing the way you feel and act in these relationships. Once you realize this, you can take that hug into the world.

What Is Hugging?

Hugging is about connection. Sometimes it's an intentional act of affection; sometimes it is more spontaneous. It doesn't have to be physical or spoken; it may just be understood. A hug is every way that you reach out and open yourself up, planned or unplanned, and share a moment or more of connection.

WHAT IS A "HUG"?

A hug can mean anything from a moment of recognition between two people who are sharing the same experience, to an affectionate, warm embrace. Hugging is not limited to throwing your arms around someone. At the other end of the spectrum, it can be as simple as two people exchanging a look. For an instant, you both recognize that you are sharing an experience, and you connect. Consider how total strangers related to each other after 9/11. We made eye contact; we talked to people we didn't know, and would likely never see again. We understood how they felt, because it was exactly how we felt. It was magic; it was also brief. It didn't last very long, but wouldn't it have been great if it had?

NO ONE-SIZE-FITS-ALL HUG

There are different kinds of hugs, and at any time, you decide which one is appropriate, with whom, and when. There are brisk hugs, and slow hugs, affectionate hugs, and quick pat on the back hugs. Each have their own time and place. Below are a few to think more about and have in your hugging arsenal.

Connecting Hug—with someone you know very well and with whom you want to strengthen the bond between you.

Creating Hug—in which you are building a new connection.

Self-Hug—Involves having self-love, and self-discipline, being straight with yourself about what you want, and what it's going to take to get it; then acting and taking loving steps to achieve your goals.

Vulnerable Hug—allowing yourself to be open, stepping outside your comfort zone, and into the hugging zone.

Concerned Hug—tough love, such as yelling at your child to get out of the street, because a car is coming, nurturing yourself by getting up in the morning when you are committed to exercising.

Virtual Hug—a personalized hug that you express in words. It tells someone what they mean to you in a profound and heartfelt way. It requires the sender to be fully present. It's magical because the person must be fully conscious in the moment to create it, and for the recipient, feeling the power of the hug is awesome. This can occur over Skype, text, FaceTime, or other social media. Virtual hugs can also be transmitted via the old-fashioned, yet invaluable hugging modes of landlines and snail mail.

Not a Hug—a way of pushing someone away either physically or metaphorically, alienating others, closing yourself off from them. Not a hug results in often feeling separate, disconnected, or isolated. Even though you are not taking action, not a hug can be as palpable as a physical hug, and can color your entire day or sometimes much longer.

WHY THIS MATTERS

This framework of identifying the type of hug that you are engaging or not engaging in is rich. It can bridge the gap between how you are and how you want to be with refreshing simplicity and pragmatism that works.

ACTION

Are you hugging the people (literally or metaphorically) that you say you love the most? If not, what's stopping you from this expression of love? Are you holding onto a particular understanding of reality that you created and are stuck in? Did something happen in the past, and are you still living as though it is happening in the present? This is a common way that people experience their world.

Returning to the example of the birthday party—let's say that the birthday party your best friend missed was three years ago. Since that time, you've never felt quite the same about that friend. Sure, they have been there for you through the death of your aunt, and a relationship breakup. You have had many special moments, and they are great in many ways, yet there is this subtle, nagging question in the back of your mind: *Are they really there for me?* If this is not addressed with radical transparency and openness, it will act as a drain on the friendship, and on your quality of life. Be thorough in looking at the distinction between reality and your version of reality. Humans have the tendency to hold onto a grudge and be in denial about holding onto that grudge. If you really look, you will start to see this within the fabric of relationships and parts of your life with which you are not satisfied.

Radical Transparency–Truth in Love

(This is a tool that will allow you to deepen your most meaningful relationships as well as to protect and maintain them. In the event that you chose to end a relationship, it is also critical for healthy closure.)

To be clear this is not "brutal honesty." This is not about hurting yourself or anyone else; this is "truth in love." The reality is that your authenticity with yourself and those around you is valuable. This has two distinct layers: Knowing what you really want, and having the clear option to share it clearly and directly with others. This essentially means asking yourself two critical questions in any given moment: "What do I really feel in this moment?" and "What am I willing to authentically share in this moment?" This will not always be easy or feel good, but I encourage you to take a hard look at all aspects of your life, experience the transformative effects of radical transparency. Consider, radical transparency can set us free, and it occurs in the space of a hug.

Let's say that your sister calls and you answer the phone, and you don't really feel like talking. Taking a moment to notice why you don't feel like talking, and assessing your current vs.

desired connection could impact how the call proceeds. A radically transparent initial statement would be, "I answered the phone, but I don't really feel like talking." This allows her to know your experience (in the moment), and proceed from that space. You may choose to talk to her for any number of reasons, and the way you feel about talking may shift; or you may decide this isn't the best time to talk. If you decide not to talk, you can communicate how important your sister is to you, so that she doesn't take your unwillingness to chat personally. This would be an example of the virtual hug that I mentioned earlier. Either option is a good one, and now you are making the decision whether or not to remain on the phone with your sister, who is likely more connected to you because you were radically transparent. The alternative is to not answer the phone, not express how you are feeling, and to create distance or increase the distance from her. Sometimes, we also answer and pretend to listen, when really not being present at all. Then, when we get off the phone, we wonder why we wasted five minutes of both our lives hiding and being false. Notice when you are on the phone with someone, and not really listening, or hoping the call will end. Who is this really serving?

Another example would be when a friend does something that upsets us, and we say nothing. Inside we may be thinking "how could they do that to me?" Or "what the F is wrong with them?" Far too often, on the outside, we just smile, nod, and act like nothing is wrong. This has many negative impacts. It doesn't allow for the friend to know what really matters to us, and it leaves us stuck in a world where disappointment is an expectation. Here is one concrete scenario that can help to explain this: Let's say that when you meet a friend for dinner and a movie, he parks his expensive new car really far away from the restaurant. You see them parking, and you walk over—perhaps looking forward to a hug. As they walk toward you, they're snarling, "Some asshole will probably park right next to me anyway, they always do." Being radically transparent would entail saying what you experience in that moment.

If this bothers you or makes you feel less connected to this friend you might say, "I felt uncomfortable when you said that. I felt like you were angry at me." The point isn't specifically what is said in this example, what matters is how you notice yourself feeling in that moment. This allows the friend the opportunity to deal with the impact their behavior has on your experience, and gives you both the possibility of learning more about one another and growing closer. Often, what happens is that rather than practicing radical transparency, we keep quiet about our feelings in a situation like this, and as a result, we can spend the whole movie frustrated about the experience, and may become less likely to spend time with this friend in the future.

Why do we hold back our true feelings and become dishonest with ourselves and the people around us? Some might say it's to protect us from things we can't or don't want to hear. Others, if truly transparent with themselves, can acknowledge that they don't know, and sometimes don't take much responsibility for what they say. Not being authentic with ourselves and with the world is not the space of a hug. Misleading ourselves or others to minimize pain is often shortsighted. We do it more to make ourselves comfortable in the moment, and to avoid growth and the unknown. The space of a hug is not always easy or comfortable.

Let's continue to explore radical transparency. The ways we mislead ourselves occur on so many levels, and become so comfortable, that we can lose sight of the truth. Marie Kondo's book *The Life-Changing Magic of Tidying Up* is delightful and has many brilliant concepts. It is well worth reading. The one message I found most riveting was the concept of holding something, and if it brings a feeling of joy, keeping it, and if not, getting rid of it. She explains that by keeping an object that doesn't bring us joy, we are surrounding ourselves with negative energy.

WHY THIS MATTERS

Clutter in our mind is no less of an issue. Share yourself with others genuinely and fully, leaving room for energy and thoughts that bring you joy.

Something similar happens when we fool ourselves or others. Consider that anytime we aren't radically transparent there is a cost. It may be subtle, and we might not feel the weight of it in that moment. Each of these little false truths constricts our world, and detracts from our connection to those we love and care about.

ACTION

Be radically transparent. Let those around you know this is something that you are dedicating yourself to. Let them know that by being authentic and honest with them, regardless of the potential discomfort of the truth in the moment—your intention is to truly share yourself with them. Sharing with them is the space of a hug. It will deepen and transform how you experience the world. Experiment with it, and test the results. Consider that radical transparency has the power to literally "set us free" in any moment that we utilize it. Truth in love.

Sphere of Hugging

There are three levels of hugging: the space of a hug, the physical hug, and the virtual hug.

The space of a hug is the ability to be with another person in a way that you each feel accepted, loved, and connected. This person may be anyone, from a stranger in the checkout line to a dear friend. There may be no physical contact at all. Nonetheless, because you are in that space, both of you will feel the effects, and the other person may experience healing or empowerment. At this moment, you are living in alignment with your deepest values.

The space of a hug is brilliant. To be truly and deeply connected with someone doesn't require any physical contact. Listening from your heart to their heart and feeling the deep human connection is sufficient. And yet, you still have two additional powerful, useful, and distinct options in your arsenal—the actual hug and the virtual hug.

VIRTUAL HUGS

What is a virtual hug? This covers a lot of ground. In a nutshell, it is any time you intentionally hug someone with the use of language, whether written, spoken, or via your phone or computer.

I notice this in the world when I feel a connection to a stranger. At the end of our exchange, I ask if they would like a hug. If they decline, I say to them something like, "I'm sending you a virtual hug with lightness and joy." Then, I will add in a piece that is fun or serious that fits with my experience of connecting with them. I may say that I hope or believe the rest of their day will be increasingly peaceful based on the virtual hug or include virtual candies and fresh, virtual chocolate-chip cookies. My focus remains on being authentic, connected, playful, and fully present in the moment. It is also modeling the power and fun of spreading virtual hugs.

A more serious instance is when, as a therapist, I feel a deep connection with someone, and they have been working with me for an extended period, sometimes a virtual hug seems a great way to express my support and unconditional love for the individual without physical touch. I'm thinking, for example, of a female client with whom I had worked for over a year, and had a positive therapeutic relationship with. One of her primary issues was that she was sexually assaulted. I was extra aware of her boundaries, and did not want to make her feel uncomfortable. In this instance, I didn't think a physical hug was appropriate, and I expressed that I was sending her a hug with my words. Although she might have liked a hug, I erred on the side of caution. It's critical to be mindful that a hug never cause the other person any harm. Sometimes, when one offers a virtual hug, the individual in question will indicate they prefer a real hug. In some ways, the virtual hug can also be a way of checking in. Of course, the individual who offers the virtual hug can choose to stick with the virtual hug if that seems the most appropriate.

Essentially, you need to meet the other person where they are. If you say, "Would you like a hug?" and you think they are saying no, verbally or nonverbally, then pass. It's often best to start with friends and family to get a feel for which types of hugging work best and why. This is a nuanced process that will unfold throughout our lives.

Although virtual hugs are a different animal than physical hugs, they are both powerful and have distinct benefits. One of the biggest obstacles to living a created/inspired life is the automatic nature of modern existence. Start to put the way you express your love for your family and friends under scrutiny. Too often, we rush goodbyes and tell the people who are most important to us that we love them without being present. The power of a virtual hug is that you are reminded to create something that requires you to be present in the moment, and wouldn't happen if you didn't create it. It's a way to express your love, your joy, your passion, and your creativity.

For example, I often send hugs with lightness and joy. However, the minute that I start saying this in a rote way without being present, I'm in automatic mode. Once this automaticity slips in, it's important that we notice it. The person I'm speaking to *may* still value what I'm saying, but I'm not really fully present. Once lightness and joy are coming out of my mouth, and I'm thinking about my next Facebook post or where to go for dinner, I'm clearly not present. The journey is about making that hug, in that moment, something that has all our attention. This may be by phone message or text or messenger, or any stated, typed, or other mode. The key is that the sender is focused on being fully present, creating that message in a way in which the sender feels alive and connected. The virtual hug is a way of dancing with life.

For example, for my sister, I will send her a hug with lightness, joy, possibilities, and a Mandelbrot. This is a dessert bread that we both know and cherish from our childhood. The point is to tailor the hug and leave it for them in a way that leaves them touched, moved, and maybe even inspired. Now, Mandelbrot was special the first time I send it, but if I'm always sending that, then it becomes rote as well. Often, if I find myself in automatic mode, I add in some sparkle on the end, such as lemon drops, light breezes, or whatever spark I feel in the moment. The key is to create it as play, dance, make yourself chuckle, crack them up, be real. Through this, they will *know* how important you are to them, and that you are giving them 100 percent of your attention and love. Don't overthink it. Let go. Know yourself to be expressing what they really mean to you; by doing this, you will feel connected to yourself in the moment, and to positivity about what you are bringing into the world.

WHY THIS MATTERS

People tend to be self-focused. When you become aware of the way you are in the world—the impact you can have moment to moment—you will allow yourself moments of exhilaration and joy.

ACTION

Envision that we have a bubble around us that touches everything we touch. This sphere is the way we connect or not with the world. For instance, let's say that you are walking through the airport, rolling your carry-on behind you. Now, you notice that a man has his hands really full with three bags and a baby. The baby is adorable, and you are taking it all in, observing the challenge for him of handling all those things and admiring how cute the baby is. When you look down at your ticket, you notice that you were so caught up in people watching that you are close to missing your flight. You start to dash off in the direction of your gate, and you notice that the baby's adorable shoe just fell off, and no one noticed. Stopping for that moment and making sure the little one gets back the shoe is a part of your Hugging Sphere. By doing this, you are in the space of a hug. Is it a big deal that the baby gets back the shoe? Not really. Likely, he or she has many other shoes, and isn't even walking yet after all. What matters here in a profound way is two things: First, you know yourself to be somebody who cares about fellow humans, and the parent (and child) in that moment know that people care about and are connected to them. It's that simple. Know yourself in each moment to be someone who chooses to connect with and empower humanity. The levels of impact humans have in the world are only limited by our imagination and investment.

Today, who can your sphere touch in your immediate vicinity and around the world?

Hug Today: This Is It—No Regrets

Live in the now. Live today fully. Let this really sink in and wash over you. Consider that there are no do-over days. Any stranger that you don't reach out to is a lost connection. Anything that you don't express to your loved ones never gets said. Don't hear this as pressure to get it right or a burden to live in a certain way. Hear this as permission to fully be you—the you that knows how much you love your mom and really wants her to know, right now; the you that wants to have a longer hug and really get lost in that hug with your friend or family member. We are promised nothing. Any of us can have a heart attack in the next moment, mid-sentence while reading. As we are all too familiar, there could be an earthquake, terrorist attack, or some other abrupt end to life. Don't let this get you down. This is the existential power to be fully connected to yourself and to the world and have a profound awareness of everything. Use this to energize yourself about *today* and express yourself fully. As my mom used to tell me, "If not now, when?"

Let's look at a few instances that you may bump up against or have already.

Perhaps there is something you really want—such as a raise or a date—but it is risky to ask for it, so you put it off. You tell yourself it isn't the right time, your boss isn't in a good mood today, that special someone will never say yes, or you haven't built your case yet.

Remember all the other times you wanted to do or say something, but thought, *Oh, I'll do it later when I've had a chance to think it through*? When later comes, you may or may not do what you planned. Either way, you've missed your moment. That moment will never come again.

You only have this moment—right now. When it's over, it's gone forever. Waiting to make a move when it feels right, or you have it all figured out is often as good as never doing it. Whatever it is, do it now, because you are not preparing for some big performance. This is the only performance. You're onstage now. This is happening in real time.

WHY THIS MATTERS

It is now or never. Hug. If you're thinking, *the next time around, I can go after what I want*, stop. There is no next time around. Jump in now and take a hugging leap of faith.

Your life is made of moments. How many have you squandered? How many more will you waste by not acting here and now? What do you really want? Be radically transparent with yourself. Tied to taking these leaps that really matter to you, this muscle (so to speak) can be strengthened by meaningfully interacting with the "strangers" all around you.

I define a stranger as someone I've known in the ballpark of three to twenty minutes. With the first stranger I hugged, I was conceptualizing a dichotomy, the difference between fear and freedom. Success in life and breakthroughs are all about going outside your comfort zone. This includes making choices about who you talk to and when.

For example, imagine that we're in line at the airport, waiting for a plane. We don't know each other, but we strike up a conversation. It's small talk. Where are you going? Do you live here? Are you going to visit family? I ask if you want a hug. I mention the power of twenty-one-second hugs, and you can decide whether you want a hug at all, and if so, for how long.

Let's say you say yes. I give you a hug, we both get on the plane, and we never see each other again. But that's okay. I stepped outside my comfort zone and did what I felt moved to do. It was a moment in time—a connection, however brief. And I would say it was more than okay on many levels. I can't be sure exactly how the other person felt unless I ask, and they tell me with radical transparency. This is what I do know: I feel good. I'm glad I had a hug and had the chance to connect in a powerful way with a fellow human. I leave that space knowing myself to be living in a connected and loving world. I also strongly believe that the people who saw us connecting felt something positive as well. It may be very subtle, but our embrace impacts them in a positive way, just like yelling or fighting with a stranger would impact them negatively. They are in the space of a hug, and I believe this, although a bit like a subliminal message, has a powerful impact. Imagine that if in this moment all over the world there were one million twenty-one-second hugs happening—physical hugs, as well as hugs for charities, kindness, and beyond. I believe, in our heart of hearts, this is the world we all want to live in. If you don't feel comfortable with a hug, if you say no, that's also totally okay. I expressed myself genuinely and let you know how I felt. You were radically transparent with me, and I consider your being truthful, and creating boundaries that work for you a self-hug.

ACTION

Before you can make any significant change in your life, you need to do three simple (but not easy) things:

Have awareness and clarity of what you are doing now.

Decide if and how you want to change that behavior.

Take action!

Once you know that you are postponing decisions or actions for some unspecified time in the future, you can decide to stop waiting. There is no perfect time to confront a tough issue, speak your mind, or ask for something important to you. Of course it feels risky or you wouldn't have put it off. Everything in life involves risk, so take a deep breath and leap. Yes, leap.

If it helps, start small with manageable challenges and build up to the bigger ones. Commit to taking at least one leap today—one you wouldn't have taken before reading this section. Think of that leap as a self-hug, regardless of the result. You will feel more alive as you take it, and know you are truly experiencing a delicious taste of what is possible. Let the adventure begin.

Planning Your 21-Day Hugging Journey

Okay, you think this 21-Day Hugging Journey has potential, and you want to give it a go, and yet, you're still asking, "what does this really look like or mean for me specifically?" That's the perfect question to be asking. Here is the answer. What do you really want in your life? Or perhaps, what do you feel you really need the journey to look like to get you unstuck or moving. All of us can use a tool to deepen our connections to ourselves and others.

The 21-Day Hugging Journey is broken down into three different parts (embrace yourself, embrace life, embrace others) to help you to figure this out. That being said, trust yourself. Perhaps, as you have been reading up to this point, you have had some thoughts, nagging questions, or a vision of what you want. Listen closely to yourself, consider that you already know. What needs to be done? What have you been putting off? It might seem scary or overwhelming. Trust you can do this, and have lots of fun along the way. All of these "little voices" are guideposts for planning your 21-Day Hugging Journey. You might be saying "I haven't heard any voices?" Don't worry. It will all be laid out as we move forward together. What comes next is a Hugging Life Snapshot to give you an overview of what parts of your life are working well, and which ones you may want to focus on or enhance.

For those of you who are raring to go at this point, here are the hugging action steps. Whether you want/need to read on a bit more, or want to jump into hugging action, have faith and trust your instincts letting this process unfold.

ACTION STEPS TO STARTING YOUR 21-DAY HUGGING JOURNEY

Declare in this moment that you are starting your 21-Day Hugging Journey today and state an intention or goal. This may be as simple as "I am going on a 21-Day Hugging Journey to create more adventure in my life, be closer to my family, be more fit, or be happier at my job." This doesn't limit you to any one area. It gives you energy to start to discover what you will create. Don't get hung up on getting the intention correct; be in action about starting *now*. You may choose to do this on social media or however feels most meaningful and supports your goals.

Now create an overview of some concrete actions and plans you have for the next 21 days and put them on your calendar for each of the next 21-days. (See Parts II, III, IV, and V)

Determine who you want to be your hugging accountability buddy and reach out to them later today or contact them right now. You don't have to have a hugging accountability buddy, although it is highly recommended.

This is a powerful tool to keep you grounded, focused, and present with consistency on your journey. If you aren't able to find a hugging accountability buddy, reach out to Hugging Central.

Complete the Hugging Life Snapshot: Day Zero

Look at the following domains and rate them on a scale of one to seven in your life today. Seven represents that this area of your life is going extremely well; it means you feel at peace in this area and feel confident you are moving in the right direction. On the other end of the spectrum, a 1 means that you are extremely disappointed with this part of your life, and it weighs on you in a very painful way on an almost daily basis. This is a snapshot to better understand where you view yourself currently, and a tool to understand how and where you might be beating yourself up, and not giving yourself a hug of forgiveness. The lines next to the rating are for you to explain why you chose this rating so that you can better understand what moving in the direction of a seven would look like. This will also be valuable when you look back in three weeks and compare your HUGGING LIFE SNAPSHOT Day Zero to your HUGGING LIFE SNAPSHOT Day 22. It will allow you to take a concrete look at your 21-Day Hugging Journey, what you created, and give you clarity about what else you might choose to delve into on a future Hugging Journey.

Below the blank ratings scale is a hypothetical example of how you might complete the list to help you proceed or to use as a reference. As in the example below, often it is valuable to give some explanation about why you chose that particular rating and to flesh out your rating for yourself. If you gave yourself a 3.5, explain what a 7 would look like in that domain and how you would know when you were at a 5, 6, or 7.

This is a powerful tool to help determine what you will choose to focus on in your 21-Day Hugging Journey. You may start off with a 21-Day Hugging Journey focused on your health, and after completing that journey and learning valuable lessons, you may choose a second journey on being closer to your mom and embracing your job. Have faith in 21-day hugging journeys unfolding organically.

At this point, it may be tempting to keep reading and tell yourself that you will do the ratings later, or that you are too busy to do a 21-Day Hugging Journey right now. As I'm writing this section, it's the day after Thanksgiving and it's a busy time with lots of holiday preparations. My point is that we often feel too busy, and can easily come up with many reasons to not pursue something. Failure to act keeps us stuck. The challenge in *this* moment is to use the power of your words to commit to a 21-Day Hugging Journey. Consider saying out loud to yourself, or to a friend, spouse, or whomever you are with, "I am going to start a 21-Day Hugging Journey today." There really is no other time to start. Too many things that really matter to us keep getting put off.

Hug Therapy is a concrete game plan to live a more meaningful, loving, and connected life. *Don't put it off.* Give yourself the hug of actively creating what you want, and know what really matters to you. Start to "hug-storm" your plan and take concrete steps to create it. It doesn't matter where you are in life. You might be a fortune 500 CEO or someone who doesn't have their own home. You might have a terminal disease or be in outstanding physical health. You might be happily married or feel bitter about your divorce. Wherever you are, whatever is happening in your life, this is a tool to support you, inspire you, and allow you to embrace life. Let the 21-Day Hugging Journey begin. Do these ratings *now*.

1. *Health Rating =* _____

   _____

   _____

   _____

2. *Family Rating =* _____

   _____

   _____

   _____

3. *Career Rating =* _____

   _____

   _____

   _____

4. *Personal Development Rating =* _____

   _____

   _____

   _____

5. Friends Rating = _____

_____

_____

_____

6. Finances Rating = _____

_____

_____

_____

7. Spiritual Development Rating = _____

_____

_____

_____

8. Intimacy Rating = _____

_____

_____

_____

9. Self-Care Rating = _____

_____

_____

_____

10. Romance Rating = _____

_____

_____

_____

11. Fitness Rating = _____

_____

_____

_____

12. Social Rating = _____

_____

_____

_____

13. Life Purpose Rating = _____

_____

_____

_____

14. Physical Environment = _____

_____

_____

_____

Health—3.0: I don't like my thighs because they seem too big and out of proportion, and I'm worried about my lungs because I am a smoker, as well as my liver because I think I may drink too much, especially when I am worried about the two grandparents I have left and how they are getting so old and likely we don't have much time left. I am so close to them and can't really bear to think of losing them.

Family—7.0: no brainer, I'd like to spend even more time with them, and we are so close, and I feel very lucky and happy.

Career—5.5: Blessed and fortuitous on some levels, good job, pays well, solid benefits, and some flexibility with my work hours—feel good about going to work and that I am doing something meaningful, although I'm not sure it is the right career for me or my "dream job." Have been there for twelve years now and I am not sure if I am comfortable in my job or that's a rationalization, and I am actually afraid of change.

Personal Development—4.0: I try to spend some time daily gaining knowledge from audio books and NPR. Often it gets away from me, and I'd like more consistency, and to not spend so much time on what feels like busy work.

Friends—4.0: I have lost some friends that I wouldn't have expected to lose in the most recent years—just by growing apart—I don't do particularly well with long distance. I miss some of my college and high school buddies, and feel like life is moving too fast to connect, and I'm not sure if they want to reconnect as much as I do. Did go on a trip to California with a close friend, and we reconnected and had a great time.

Finances—5.0: Room to be better, but I can't complain too much—Feel good about earning and not spending, although having three kids and knowing that college is only a few years around the corner is pretty daunting. We have been saving, but still, it stresses me out a few days a week.

Spiritual Development—5.5**:** I go to church almost every Sunday. Sometimes I feel like I am just doing it because that is how I was raised. The sermon is usually meaningful, and helps me to be grateful and focus on what really matters. Not sure how I feel about God, but I do feel connected to the church and I know it grounds me. I feel like I often see the spiritual side of things and this helps me to take life in stride and remember the bigger picture.

Intimacy—5.5: Relationships with people and connections are pretty good and kind of casual; they could be deeper or more meaningful, I guess. I don't know if I really want or need that, maybe I will move this one up to a 6 or even 6.5.

Self-care—4.0: I enjoy being active and I go on hikes pretty regularly—still I know that I smoke and drink too much and that it is messing with me.

Romance—2.0: Well for where I am at in my marriage, I guess I will rate this one at a 2 even though it makes me really sad to say it. I love my wife and I feel really connected to her sometimes; at others, it feels like I just have a roommate. We have now been married for almost twelve years and sometimes I think she takes me for granted and other times she doesn't really seem to notice me, just sometimes and it hurts. I hate to think we are growing apart because I love her so much and yet I know we need to do something.

Fitness—3.0: Probably rate it this way, because I have always wanted to run a marathon and I never have. My son is an athlete and I'd like for us to train and run one together, but I've never even told him my dream and I'm not sure why. If I was in condition and training daily with him, and could actually have fun running a marathon, that would be a 7 for me. It now occurs to me that I am definitely going to talk to my son and start that conversation.

Social—6.0: I'm pretty social and I think I am easy to talk to, and I enjoy my friends and social activities, but a lot of the time I don't set anything up and I like my alone time as well.

Life purpose—5.0: Well, I go to church regularly and the sermons are meaningful to me. We give a good amount of charity and I do some volunteering. Sometimes though, I just feel like what's the point? Am I making a difference? Does

Hug Therapy

any of this really matter? I guess moving toward a 7 would be aligning what I am doing at work more with what really matters to me. Or maybe I need to start to consider other job possibilities. I'm super passionate about the charity I work with helping kids who have a parent with a drug addiction. The board did have a paid opening and I was tempted by it, but I guess scared. I need to check if that is still open and even what it pays or if they would consider me. It would be a big change, but I think it might be time for the next chapter in my life.

Physical Environment—3.0: Home is good. I'm happy in my house and I feel at peace. The big issue is work. I am in a cubicle and I have no windows. I feel like when I am there sometimes that I am like a flower that is wilting because of the artificial lights. Supposedly it is temporary, and we are going to have a state-of-the-art facility in which I will have a window with a view, but they have been talking about that for over a year now, and haven't even broken ground on the new facility. Sometimes, I just want to bang my head on my desk. I do my best to get outside and take a walk, but most of the time I am just too damn busy, and I eat lunch at my desk. I can feel my blood starting to boil as I am thinking about this, I think I need to move it down to a 2.0 or less. I mean I spend like sixty hours a week in that f*cking cubicle.

Great work. Now that you have completed your ratings you have a tool to help you to choose what you want to focus on in your first 21-Day Hugging Journey. You may pick one specific domain, such as becoming closer to your mother. You may also choose a number of domains that resonate for you, and work at improving your fitness, finances, and physical environment. The challenge is to choose what feels right to work on, right now, and do so in a way that holds you accountable and keeps you steadily moving forward. In addition, when you find you aren't making steady progress, you can refer back to these ratings to help you be radically transparent with yourself about why you might have gotten stuck, and put a plan in place to support you on the next day of your Hugging Journey.

Although each person's journey is unique to them, hopefully, it is starting to become clearer about how forgiveness or lack of forgiveness of yourself in different domains is a thread which weaves through our lives.

No matter what happened in the past, becoming more aware of your pain points can be the first step in forgiving yourself and letting go of any guilt you carry. This is not easy, and it is critical to identify that it is a choice. Maybe this means writing a letter and burning it or burying it. Maybe this means having a heartfelt conversation. Maybe this means... You decide what it will take to have some freedom from this judgment that you carry with you everywhere. This heavy weight that holds you down and stops you from being at peace with reality. Trust. Whatever you have done, it's over and it can't be changed. By definition it is your past. Clean it up with who it's impacted, and literally give yourself the joy and magic of a fresh start. Letting go of it once likely won't be the end of it, but you can give yourself a fresh start as many times as you need one.

This will show you that you can be radically transparent with yourself and deal with whatever pain you are holding onto. Likely, you will need to come back to it, and let it go again tomorrow, and continue the "hug work." Today, allow yourself the freedom and play of the purity of who you really are.

Let me explain further with a personal pain point from my life.

I'm divorced, after being married for eleven years. We have two beautiful children, but sadly the romantic love was gone from our marriage. Perhaps a century earlier we would have stayed unhappily married, because that's what people did, and sometimes still do. We chose divorce. This was extremely painful at the time, and remains sometimes painful to this day. I never intended (as I'm sure no one does) that I would end the relationship (with the then love of my life). I first really started to accept that the marriage wasn't going to work when a close friend said to me, "If she's really just a roommate, what's the point?" I didn't want to accept that my marriage might be over. I fought it hard in my mind and in my heart. Couples therapy was helpful, but no matter what we did, it didn't seem to make a real difference. I could spend more time analyzing or explaining, but the point is that I am divorced, and have been for over five years. That being said, sometimes an unhealthy view of reality can sneak up on me. It might be very subtle, and it has the flavor of "you never should have gotten divorced; life would be so much better if your family was together." Arguments could be made that my life would be better, and it would definitely be different, but the reality is that "I am divorced." Embracing that I am divorced is the starting place for moving forward and forgiving myself and/or anyone else I might blame. Could I have done some things differently or better? Certainly. Would they have changed the reality of being divorced? I will never know. Whatever it is that you have done, it is done. How will beating yourself up about it help? If this is something that you are doing, ask yourself, "how is that working for you?"

Now did I just embrace being divorced one time? Definitely not. It has been many years, and there are still times when I think "what if?" The challenge and the journey are about having awareness of what we are experiencing and embracing it in the most productive way in the present moment. I can slip into thinking, "what if I was happily married and attending various events with or spending present moments with my children?" It's okay for me to think about this and be radically transparent with myself about what thoughts and feelings are there for me, and feel the sadness or confusion. One reason that it is okay is that the alternative, to try and shut it out, really isn't effective. People often will say "I just let it roll off my back." Or perhaps, "it doesn't really phase me." In my clinical and personal experience, it impacts us in various ways, and avoiding the feelings is counter-productive, and at times, not even realistic. Sometimes people go down a slippery slope trying to avoid these feelings with alcohol, drugs, or other types of addiction.

Try for a moment, right now, not to think about a pink elephant. You might be questioning this exercise, but take a little leap of faith, and do this, even if it feels weird. Allow yourself to take a few seconds and try your very best not to think of a pink elephant. I don't want you to think about how they are usually gray and this one is pink. I don't want you to think about how it is one of the largest animals or how they have a huge trunk that can shoot water. Don't think about this. Don't think about any associations or past experiences that you have about elephants, or the zoo, or anything regarding these huge, gentle animals. How does this work for you? How are you doing with not thinking about a pink elephant?

Some might say, that was easy, I just focused on something else. I was thinking about a black limousine, my Aunt Bessie, or all the things on my to do list. I would encourage you to consider that the whole time you were attempting not to think about a pink elephant, that thought was always there just below the surface. If I told you I had a valuable prize I would give you if you could tell me what you weren't thinking of, you'd likely say pink elephant quite quickly. It's almost impossible not to experience something that we intentionally avoid.

I do my best to let myself have thoughts and feelings about my divorce. But, I also embrace and have gratitude for all of the things that are working, and for which I am grateful. My children are healthy and loved. I am able to be in new relationships, and I have freedom to do different things that really matter to me. I regularly see my children (we have joint custody), and they know how much I love them. It is often a struggle to maintain a healthy balance between allowing yourself the thoughts or feelings that may come up around loss or change, and living life now. This may be due to the death of a loved one or losing a job. The key balance to be aware of, and strive to live in, is to allow yourself to feel what is there, and not to shift into *victim mode*.

When I say planning, don't think weeks, months, or years. The idea is to jump into your journey, either right now, in the next 21 seconds, 21 minutes, and definitely within the next 21 hours. Don't get caught in planning paralysis. *Action is key.* Consider how many times we think "oh that sounds like such a good idea for me, I'll definitely do it at some point." Way too often, someday never comes, because the next responsibility or priority fills up our life and whatever we intended to do escapes our attention, often permanently. The secret here is to use the power of your words with friends, family, and on social media to declare to the world or whomever you choose "I'm going on a 21-Day Hugging Journey." Then allow yourself to create as you move forward. Yes, have a game plan. And, much of the magic comes as you move into the world in "the space of a hug."

Two key questions to ask yourself to help with clarity are: what *regrets* do I have about my life up to this point? and What do I *hate* most about my life?

Asking these questions is smart, because it gives you a brave moment to look deeply and radically transparently into your life and assess how it is and how it isn't working. Only you can do this, and it takes guts. Look from a hugging place. Don't beat yourself up or judge, simply look and see what you notice. Perhaps one of the first things that comes up is "I never call my mom and I miss her." This will guide you on how you plan the next 21-days. Your journey could be simply and powerfully focused on "getting closer to mom." That's a beautiful journey.

It is going to look different for each of us. The point is you can only get closer to her today. You can only get closer to anyone today, for that matter, today in this moment. The reality is we don't know if tomorrow you will be alive, or she will be alive. We take it for granted. Nothing is promised. That is why it's so important to start your Hugging Journey today. If you don't think you are as close as you want to be with your mom, you are the only one that can make that change. (You might be thinking "well she could reach out to me." True, and if you aren't really in the space to be more connected with her, then it likely won't mean much, more on that later.)

There are lots of different ways to be more connected to her, and it all ties into the history you have with her, and what's in the way of you two being close. What I would call the "anti-hug." One powerful way to start might be simply to reach out to her on day one, by phone, email or in person, and tell her, "I am going on a 21-Day Hugging Journey, because I want to be closer to you." You could than go on to explain that this is a hugging journey about being closer to her. You could together lay out a plan to talk every day and plan some special things over the next three weeks. You could tell her radically transparently, "I am reading this book and it's talking to me about living like tomorrow isn't promised. It made me realize I want more time with you, and I am taking action to make that happen." This is one example of how to really throw yourself into your life. Now you may be thinking of various objections like, "my mom lives in Iceland" or "I work eighty hours a week at my job." That is all relevant, and at the same time, this is where the rubber meets the road. You are way too powerful to let the relationship with your mom slip away day after day; don't fool yourself and think it's not hurting your overall quality of life. Even when you are sitting with friends in a beautiful place and enjoying life, that disconnect or lack of connection from your mom is there. It matters, and likely weighs on you. It's lurking there, just below the surface. *Hug Therapy* is here to wake you up to the reality of not waiting until it is too late.

Act while you can with your mother or anyone else you have been shortchanging. And this isn't for them, although it will have a profound impact on them, this is for you. You are the one you have been shortchanging the most. You can fill that empty space with love and connection, take action, and do what you know is right and really matters to you.

You might be saying, "but my mom died five years ago." If that is the case, I am sorry to hear of your loss. You can still have a 21-Day Hugging Journey focused on being closer to your mom and having healthy closure. Even if a parent or anyone who was a key part of our childhood has died, they can still have a huge impact. Express to them aloud or in your journal what you really want or need to say to them. Perhaps, you weren't able to be with them when they died in that last moment, and that weighs on you. Perhaps, you never got to tell them something that you really wanted them to know. Perhaps you said something to them that you have always regretted. Now is the time to write them a letter and say what you really want and need to say. Depending on your spiritual beliefs, you may believe they have an awareness of what you are communicating to them, or you may not. Trust that part of *Hug Therapy* for you is to express these doubts, these questions, these regrets, or these hopes onto paper or aloud. Your 21-day Journey may involve going to their tombstone and speaking to them. It may be setting up a charity in their name, or talking to a sibling or a dear friend about them. Anything that weighs on you, don't hold on to it, find a way to express it, and let go of the burden. This may be what you choose on your journey. Look inside and see what regrets or unfinished business can be handled, leaving you with more freedom to be fully connected and alive.

Your 21-Day Hugging Journey could also be simply and profoundly to be more connected with your spouse or romantic partner. Have you guys been slipping apart? Are they the love of your life and something feels wrong? Perhaps they aren't cuddling as much or don't seem to have time to really talk or listen to you? If this person matters to you deeply, this may be the plan for your 21-Day Hugging Journey. Maybe you've been thinking all of this, but haven't said anything aloud. It's highly unlikely that it's going to magically get better unless you take hugging action. Does this person *really* matter to you? Why not take the action to put things back on course? What is the likely future of this relationship if things keep eroding?

Be radically transparent with yourself about what actions you've taken that have caused distance. Have you made promises, such as, "we will definitely have a date this week, just the two of us" and then not kept them (a very human thing to do)? And then somebody gets sick or a big project comes up at work. Take full ownership of this with your lover, and make a commitment and a plan that really works, building trust and connection. This person loves you and is choosing to be with you. Why not be on a 21-Day Hugging Journey to make this relationship not only work, but also buzz, whir, and shine brightly?

Part of the secret is to share with others what you are up to. You don't have to. If you think "I'm a private person. I don't want others in my business." Okay. Trust that. And for some people, including introverts, consider that when you share, it can empower you, and help others to start exploring what's possible for them. The connection can enhance everything.

"What do I hate about my life?" Look hard. If the answer is nothing. Awesome. And ask the question, "what doesn't really work that well in my life?" Look deeply. Be radically transparent with yourself. If the answer is "my job," that's another important journey to embark on.

Many of us spend so much of our lives at work. Likely, the job we have is critical to how much we do or don't enjoy our lives. If you identify that you hate your job, there are lots of possibilities and ways to transform the situation. First, you have to identify what specifically it is you hate, and be radically transparent with yourself about why you are at the job. Often people are trapped by "golden handcuffs" doing a job they don't like for what they hope it will provide their family in the future. Whether or not you stay at your job or decide you want to create something different is something that will unfold over your 21-Day Hugging Journey. This may be something in your life leaving you feeling powerless and yucky. This is not a way any of us wants to live, and often drains us of energy to spread hugs and love in other areas of life.

Remember that you don't have to leave the job. You may choose to, and discover that the grass is not always greener on the other side. Keep in mind what you really want, and then you can plan how to powerfully impact your current situation. It might start with some deep self-reflection and taking responsibility for the choices that you have made up to this point. After all, no one forced you to take your current job (I imagine), and you were likely excited when you started. It will be key to finding clarity about what has changed, and then, after being radically transparent with yourself, it will likely be important to be radically transparent with your boss. If you are hating your job, it is likely impacting your work performance, and an employer will likely be open to having a conversation about how you can be happier and more productive. All of this will unfold as you continue to take action with the different components of *Hug Therapy*.

The next sections break down different ways you can engage in your hugging journey. Right now, stop for a second and take a deep breath. Consider letting go of the expectation that it has to be right, or that you have to do it in a certain way. Not at all. Give yourself the freedom to do it, how you do it. Know that the Hug Doctor is available to you, as well as a team of hugging experts, and that we are deeply invested in you getting value from your journey. So give yourself permission to jump into action. Trust in yourself and this process. Although it may feel a bit scary initially, it will likely also be exciting and fresh. The examples laid out below are designed to help you to have a launching pad to create change in your life. Create a deeply meaningful impact whether with your health, friends, family, or whatever area you choose to hug. This is a game we call life. Embrace some new rules, hug yourself, and see where it takes you. I acknowledge you in advance for your commitment to yourself and for making the "space of a hug" one that continues to grow.

Part III

Embrace Yourself

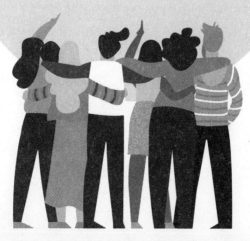

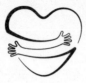

The foundation and grounding for all things that people do in the world and the way they experience themselves is tied to the self-hug. In other words, loving ourselves first. If that is not the case for you in this moment, this is something you can choose to start right now. It isn't necessary to understand why the love wasn't there in the past. Instead, begin to give yourself a hug right now. Humans by nature are whole and completely loving and accepting beings at the core. Now, today is the time to start allowing self-love to wash over you and to move forward in the space of a hug. Ask yourself: Do I love myself? What does that look like? The following are concrete examples of actions you can choose to take, demonstrating that you love yourself, based on how you are treating yourself. Even if you question your love for yourself, or you are certain that you don't love yourself, hug/step forward and let the actions create the feeling you are missing.

The other critical question is "why specifically don't you love yourself in this moment?" What belief are you holding onto that is getting in the way of you loving yourself? I would encourage you to go back and read "When All Is Said and Done."

Okay, maybe you are finding this too abstract. This is where the rubber really meets the road and radical transparency becomes key. Let's just imagine for a minute that you are sitting there thinking back to when you were fifteen years old and stole a hundred dollars from your parents. For sake of this example let's assume that this escalated over time and you stole significant sums from your family, causing financial hardship for them. These are the kinds of situations to varying degrees that we each carry. It might be that you cheated on your boyfriend or girlfriend. It may have that you cheated on an exam. It doesn't matter whether or not you got caught. It's still significant in how you see yourself, because you live with it every day. You caught you, and trust that you are punishing yourself. It may have been a major offense, such as a felony, or a smaller crime or wrongdoing.

To be clear, crystal clear, I am not condoning any abusive or unhealthy behaviors that anyone may have engaged in or committed.

Regardless of what happened, take a hard look at how punishing yourself and/or hating yourself is helping anyone. I want you to consider that not only is it not helping, it is actually exacerbating the problem for you, the person you wronged, and the world.

So, let's think back to a scenario that you may have engaged in, and feel guilty about. It is time to be radically transparent with yourself about what actually happened. What are the facts, and then, what have you been telling yourself and perpetuating since that event? *Did that really happen, and am I completely certain that actually happened?* I want you to consider whether or not you feel guilty or justified in some way that this continues to profoundly impact you each day. Once you bring these thoughts into the light, you will naturally get back in touch with how you are a natural creation, as perfect as any other part of nature. Allow yourself the freedom to begin to take care of and support yourself on a whole new level. You can choose to handle this situation in a way that moves you forward and may involve a number of conversations or actions that create freedom.

Next, I provide lots of ways to court yourself and show yourself the love you deserve!

Self-Hug

Hug yourself right now, long and hard, for a minimum of twenty-one seconds. This may be something you have never done, something that puts you outside your comfort zone. It doesn't matter if you're in a public place and worry people might laugh or stare. Hugging yourself is a way to acknowledge that you accept and believe in yourself just as you are. Without this self-acceptance, you feel incomplete, empty. Your public persona may radiate self-confidence, but deep inside, you know it's only a façade. Whatever you've done or failed to do in your life that is causing you regret, it is in the past. Whatever baggage you are carrying that is weighing you down, now is the time to let it go, to forgive, and realize that, at this moment, you are whole and complete.

So, hug yourself; fully embrace the essence of who you are. Let this hug from you, for you, wash over and help you move forward in your life. There's no time like the present, so do it today. Do it right now.

WHY THIS MATTERS

While it's great to have the approval and affection of others, the most important hug you will ever get is from yourself. Regardless of what you consider your failures, successes, or false starts so far, you can create a new start. From this point on, you can realize your own strengths, accept your weaknesses, and begin again. Only you can do this; no one can do it for you. Change your paradigm and create a new life, or continue to let the past weigh you down. This is one of those things that, although simple, can be very challenging and at first feel foreign and uncomfortable. It takes increased awareness and commitment to loving yourself.

ACTION

Ask yourself some tough questions. What did you do that is worth a lifetime of self-recrimination? Or perhaps, what did someone else do that you can't forgive? Did this event happen when you were a child, or more recently? What is getting in the way of living life to the fullest? Although this is a straightforward concept, people hold on to their past, sometimes for decades. This is not a onetime activity. You can find value in it again and again.

Take a long, hard look at the facts, whatever they are. Write them down. Try to recall what happened—not the story you tell yourself, but the truth, as close as you can come to it.

It might look like this with the following example: My best friend didn't come to my birthday party three years ago. She said that she wasn't feeling well that night, and then took me out to dinner a few nights later. She had recently gone through a relationship breakup, and was struggling with ending an unhealthy relationship.

What meaning did I create from this incident? Maybe I can't trust her, and she isn't really there for me. I took it as a personal affront. But I never said anything to her, and yet I know it makes me feel less connected to her.

The truth is that she missed one event, and she communicated that she needed to miss it. I found this painful, but I never addressed it with her, and over the past three years, I have been looking for any evidence to support my assumption that she isn't a good friend.

Does this example feel familiar? Are you thinking of a family member or friend you've had a similar distancing experience with, and the weight of it is something that you try to ignore? Life is too short. Pay close attention to the next chapter. You don't need to continue to carry this weight around with you. Clean this type of relationship up so that you can use your energy for what matters, instead of being a victim to stories from the past that you and waste precious time and energy justifying and defending.

The following sample exercises involve Embracing Yourself. The ways that you choose to embrace yourself may include these, and may also be completely different. Look at your life, allow yourself to connect with what would be nourishing for you and how you can most effectively take action to incorporate this healthy activity. When creating these exercises, the goal was to make them as valuable as possible. The objective was to avoid being trite, and instead to use deepest life regrets and what is currently deeply upsetting you as a gauge for where to start. Being radically transparent about these aspects of life provides the foundation for you to take responsibility for all parts of your life and then create powerfully. Consider you have a choice about the way you relate to these regrets and pain points and your relationship to the parts of your life that cause suffering.

Some of the exercises may seem basic at first glance. Consider that if you delve in deeply, they will have a powerful impact, sometimes quite quickly. Be careful not to disregard anything prematurely simply because it appears to be familiar, easy, or too basic. Allow these exercises to stimulate your creativity, and be responsive to how they speak to you. Your feedback is greatly appreciated and may be included in future editions of *Hug Therapy*.

Forgive Yourself

Consider that it is in our makeup to beat ourselves up, and that this is subtly tied to our survival mechanism. When we take an inventory, we'll find that there are many things that we judge ourselves for, and that weigh on us heavily. Sometimes we become so used to carrying these burdens we often don't even notice. Gaining access to these spots that are subtly or not so subtly holding us back and sucking the joy out of life is critical to the forgiveness process. This is an opportunity to look deeply at what has happened in the past, for example, a divorce, family struggle, or relationship breakup, and begin to let it go. Consider that holding on to it is like standing in a scalding hot shower and pretending that your skin isn't blistering and in pain. This is how we often live our lives. This is an important time to be radically transparent with yourself, and with others in your life to better understand what you have and what you want. Below are a few hypothetical examples of people showing what they might focus on for their 21-day hugging journeys. These were created to give you a better sense of what others might choose to focus on. Some of the dynamics may also resonate for you specifically or remind you of something else valuable for your journey.

Franky Lee (LGBT), sixty years old, is a self-made man who created his own clothing line. He is an extremely likable people person, who has a tendency to put others first, and not to make enough time for himself. Franky Lee deeply values his connection with people, and goes out of his way to help others to a fault. He believes in a world that works for everyone, is frustrated that he doesn't spend more time working on this bigger picture, and feels trapped by his business. He also has significant trouble with delegating, which is tied to trust issues. Franky Lee has been in a relationship with his romantic partner, William, for twenty-five years, and this is the only person he truly trusts. William is the love of his life, and Franky Lee also struggles to balance the demands of work with being available in his personal life. He may take significant time off for vacations, etc. at the chiding/demanding of William, but Franky Lee is always at the office to some extent. He just can't seem to disconnect from work, and this causes growing strain with William.

Fundamental Complaint/Pain Point: lack of energy, feeling down, worried about his legacy

21-Day Hugging Journey possibility for Franky Lee is to be more connected and romantic with his partner, and for them to work together to create healthy boundaries from work. This might involve possibly calling in an outside consultant. An overarching focus for Franky Lee is strengthening his ability to ask for help, learning to say no, and making this a goal for each day on his journey. His partner William could potentially be his hugging accountability buddy, or it could be someone else Franky Lee feels would be most effective in helping him to set firm and healthy limits. He can start to brainstorm about how to creative healthy boundaries to prevent his work life bleeding into his personal life.

Jane Johnson (JJ), fifty years old, is a business owner, who doesn't have a relationship with her mother, and this is something she carries with her every day. If things stop right now, she will go to her deathbed having felt her life was wasted. Without the connection to, and validation of her mother, everything else is going through the motions. On the surface, both personally and professionally, JJ is in total control, including her finances and personal life. At times, the level of control that she commands can cause strain with her children and husband. On the surface, and in many tangible ways, her life is working. She is a great mother, a loving wife, and a successful business owner, but underneath is distraught that she doesn't have a relationship with her mother, and this feels hopeless to her.

Fundamental Complaint/Pain Point: sense of emptiness, feels she is living a lie

JJ declares on day 1 of her hugging journey, "I want to be close with my mother and forgive her and myself for everything that has happened." JJ could write a long letter of her fears, her regrets, and her sadness that she could then share with her husband, who is largely in the dark about her pain, and stop living the lie that everything is okay. Together with her husband, she can start to figure out how to best approach her mom and/or consider if that makes sense. She might choose to go to therapy to better understand her childhood; she might choose to visit her mom out of state; she might start a hobby that connects her more to her mother. She can start to take action about what really matters to her. No matter what happens with her mother, she will no longer be living a lie, and will have a chance to become closer with her mother before it is too late.

Rich Artisan, forty-seven years old, is an artist and hairstylist, who has had moderate success, and is struggling to find balance. He has a certain energy about him that is contagious, and his personality is quite charming. What he secretly dreams about is being a musician. His older brother died in a car accident, and he blames himself even though there was no connection to Rich having had anything to do with the accident. He has been in therapy multiple times, and generally finds therapists to be removed and uncaring. He uses this lack of connection with past therapists to confirm his thought, "I don't really need therapy." Yet, he stays up late at night writing music, and is completely at peace with the world when he is playing his guitar and thinking about his lost brother. He is afraid to take his music to another level, even though friends and colleagues tell him he has a gift. When pushed, he will say "I really don't want to be in the spotlight." Secretly, he knows this is a huge lie, and simply put, he is afraid. To overcome this fear, he has thrown himself into the personal growth arena and has attended four different weekend workshops. These deeply resonate for him, and yet, he is struggling to bring them into his life, and take meaningful action. He's always chasing the next thing, and lacks continuity.

Fundamental Complaint/Pain Point: Self-doubt and loneliness

Rich's 21-Day Hugging Journey might involve him having an unveiling of his brother's grave or another commemorative ceremony. Perhaps one in which he writes a special song for his brother that shares his heartache and pain about the loss. He never attended the funeral, and he has never forgiven himself for this decision. At the time, he was overwhelmed with grief, and didn't leave his house for close to a week, and struggled intensely with suicidal thoughts. For 21 days Rich can commit to talking with a family or friend about his brother, and possibly raise money for a cause that was deeply meaningful to his brother.

Paul Bunyan is an introvert, but has forced himself to be an extrovert to be successful in his business. This leaves him emotionally drained, and many times seeking to escape people. This is very confusing to others, because they have no idea he is an introvert. At times he can be full of himself. This is partly due to him being a gifted athlete and very bright. He is secretly furious that he isn't a professional athlete.

He believes that, regarding his family or his business, he always has the right answer, and he rarely listens to others. He often won't even pretend to listen. Handsome and sweet to others in clutch moments, he is able to get away with this to an extent, but he pays a heavy toll over time. Paul is very successful on the surface, including financially, and feels a deep emptiness that he goes to great lengths to avoid. When he starts to feel a hint of his frustration with his friends and family, he beats this emptiness aside through intense physical activity. (He's recently taken up marathons and is training for his second.) He doesn't enjoy running, and sees it as a punishment, because he hasn't achieved his dream of being a professional athlete, and is living what he considers to be a lie. He deeply loves the people in his life, but is terrible at showing or expressing affection. This particularly leaves his children doubting themselves and their relationship to him, and they desperately seek his approval. The result is disconnection, and he is frustrated in his attempts to understand how others treat him and why they are so "needy." He is driven by forces outside of his control that he is afraid to look at; he keeps his focus on maintaining the façade that everything is "fine."

Fundamental Complaint/Pain Point: Self-focused, limited insight, difficulty communicating his true feelings to those he loves

Paul's is one of the toughest 21-day hugging experiences to predict. He knows that he is miserable, and he isn't that clear about why. If he looks at his life through a radically transparent

Hug Therapy

lens, he might choose to open up and discover what's not working for him. If he is brave enough to look at his pain and recognize that he is punishing himself, he could choose to open up to one key person in his life, perhaps his spouse, best friend, or a therapist, or coach. He could slowly look at what he can genuinely enjoy in life, and start to forgive those he blames for not becoming a pro-athlete, including himself.

Surprise and Delight Yourself Today

One of the critical challenges in life that has been alluded to throughout the book is having enhanced awareness of monotony or routine. Otherwise, the tendency is to sleepwalk through life and not take full advantage of the present moment. The "self-hug" part of the journey is about looking deeply at what you really want, and then allowing yourself the space to create. This involves a discovery process and it is often about the "little things." Yet, are they really little at all? These are the things that have an impact of major magnitude on us over time. The things that might escape us if we didn't look closely, and yet these are the life moments that, piece by piece (hug by hug), make up the fabric and quality of our lives.

On this part of the journey, do what it takes to remind yourself and be powerfully in touch with your aliveness. This is designed to be the complete opposite of "going through the motions." What are the actions (maybe ones you have been thinking about for a long time) that will show you with laser clarity how much *you* love you? Consider as you plan for your hug journey, what is something special that you want to do for you and have been putting off? This might be a fishing trip; it might be a pedicure; it might be a walk on the beach. This is your chance to take a hard look at what would surprise and delight you, and then either do it today, or in this moment. Take action to schedule it, so that it will occur on your 21-Day Hugging Journey.

One example of this is happened on day 10 of my hugging journey. I was in Boulder, CO, to visit my cousin and meet his fiancé. Because I was on a hugging journey, I was choosing to embrace life. It was a beautiful sunny day in Boulder, and I was walking to a yoga class. However, it had snowed a good deal the few days before, and everything was melting. It was to my great surprise, and not delight, when I jumped over some muddy water to a patch of snow. I found my entire foot, up to my ankle, completely soaked in slush. It was freezing, and I still had about half a mile to walk. At first, I think I cursed, and then I considered turning back, getting changed, and missing my yoga class with my cousin. Reminding myself that I was on a hugging journey, I consoled myself; I wasn't actually hurt, nor in any danger. I rolled up my pant leg and removed my soaked sock. I did my best to dry my soaked leg, put my clog type shoe back on, and I kept going. I started to realize that although jarring, and not my first choice, the cold air on my bare left foot was invigorating. It made me more aware of my surroundings, and kept me engaged in the moment. Part of surprising and delighting ourselves is discovering how we can gracefully embrace situations that are challenging, unexpected and, as we all know, a big part of life.

I am often surprised and delighted by how reaching out to people whom I don't know results in a positive impact on the world. I am often pleasantly shocked or surprised by what we have in common and that we share similar goals or values. Much of the time, I feel more connected to people in general and positive about humanity. This may be something that surprises and delights you as well. Regardless, make it a priority each day to discover who and what is around you, so that you can be surprised and delighted.

The other important thing is that I didn't let that soaked and unexpected slush experience stop me from what mattered. I made it to the yoga class, which was amazing, and stayed on track to spend quality time with my cousin.

Later that night, still on my hugging journey, and still having room to be surprised and delighted, I was walking in the snow, amazed by the beauty and the size of the snowflakes. I met a couple of sisters and their friend walking, and started to talk to them about my hugging journey, and the power of hugging. If you want to see the video go to the Hug Doctor website. It is day 10 of my Facebook Live journey. I begin talking to strangers at about 1 minute and 45 seconds into the video, and the entire clip is about 6 minutes.

You will hear me talking about the book as "Hugging Strangers" because that was the original working title before it was transformed into *Hug Therapy*. For those of you who are unable or don't want to connect to the internet, the upshot is that in Boulder, on day 10 of my Hugging Journey, I run into two sisters and their friend Christian while I am live on Facebook. I tell them about 21-second hugs and the hugging movement as we are all standing outside on Pearl Street with huge snowflakes falling all around us. First, the sisters have a hug, and then Christian joins in, and I do as well. I explain to them a little bit about hugging journeys and I am surprised and delighted as I am reminded that my strength in the belief that "there really are no strangers" is powerfully confirmed.

Fitness, Fitness, Fitness

A medical doctor once told me "if you don't use it you lose it." A critical component of a self-embrace is self-care, which includes being fit in a way that works for you. This is a daily challenge, commitment, and/or reality for each of us.

This and our diets are two things we are bombarded with messages about through the media and our social interactions. The beauty of the 21-Day Hugging Journey is that it allows us to look closely at what we are currently doing regarding fitness, and how well this is, or isn't working, in our lives. Many people have high expectations for being fit, and then don't meet those expectations, leaving them feeling frustrated and confused. This can result in "beating oneself up," and feeling like a failure in that circumstance. Beating oneself up is the exact opposite of a hugging journey's essence. This journey full of self-hugs is about loving oneself, regardless of failed attempts in the past, or of being at any current level of physical conditioning. It's about living in *this* moment and having gratitude for your current body in the "self-hug space." Then you can move forward with continued or increased fitness as you choose. Perhaps you have always wanted to take tennis lessons and now you can give yourself that hug. Maybe you have a close friend who is taking up biking, and you can reach out to them to share in that experience. What can make your fitness something that you enjoy that isn't a burden or heavy weight? How can you think outside of the box (say doing yoga each night for five minutes before bed)? Whatever you can do, embrace yourself and set yourself up for success. This is a sense of what hugging yourself looks like in the land of fitness. What if you plan to run tomorrow and oversleep? It happens. In the space of a hug acknowledge that you missed one day. Next, put steps in place, maybe contacting your hugging accountability buddy and seeing if they want to join you for a jog the next day, so that you are in action, and know yourself to be someone who is loving and gracious to yourself in a way that works in this moment and supports fitness going forward.

My dear friend Theo Lewis Clark completed a 21-Day Hugging Journey and he called it his "Journey back to Me." His focus throughout the journey was on self-care, loving himself, and making his health the top priority. He shared with me daily about his fitness routine, the additional hugs he was having, and how he felt more connected. I responded to him with consistent support and reminded him he is a leader and that his actions are powerful.

These are some of his texts. "*Day 4 of my 21-Day Journey back to me.* I still made it to the gym at six this morning and added two machines @ 4 sets of 15 to my workout. I'm also meeting with an engineer to help with my 2 upcoming radio shows! I'm also going to introduce him to my former partner who will need his skills as he starts Dynasty Television Radio. What a 4th day hug!!!"

"Day 7… ON my way to church for the first time in months!! HALLELUJAH"

"Day 8…Grateful to be strong enough to go into the gym to lift (being super consistent) and I'm going to be on the microphone today in the EG radio studios with some more cool friends, Scott and Shoe, who care about helping me have a great syndictable radio show! 8 also happens to be the number of new beginnings. Wow!"

"Day 13… On my way to a rare Saturday weightlifting session and then to Starbucks to further prepare for Monday's very important recording session."

"Day 14… I helped my sister move two couches to my niece's home. Now I'm at Starbucks enjoying a coffee while working on my show so tomorrow's recording session goes as great as possible!"

"Day 18… After learning some very bad news yesterday I got up anyway and went to the gym had a great workout, took a friend to lunch, then he and I washed my vehicle, now I'm on the way to a business meeting to uncover synergistic opportunities."

"Day 19… I love giving back to the young have nots and an influential person in the marketplace met me to talk about his similar vision to help the kids."

"Day 20… Me and my dad got to spend "quality time" day where we wake up early go run errands and laugh and talk. When we were at Walmart he commenced to throwing up and the paramedics came to take him to the hospital. That wake-up call of fathoming having him not be around, ignited an appreciation and a gratefulness I thought was already at max capacity. God is good my dad is resting comfortably."

"Day 21… Feb 5th. Five is the number of grace and God's grace is sufficient and merciful. He's had mercy on me, and he's given me joy unspeakable. This has been the fastest 21-days in my life and it's helped solidify what I know to be true. Life is short, serve somebody and have pure joy! Thanks Dr. Stone."

Theo used connecting with me by text on a daily basis as a way to keep himself grounded and meaningfully on track with his journey. It is key to determine the method that works best for you.

One of the most powerful methods so far has been the combination of Facebook Live and having a hugging accountability buddy. When the hugging ambassador, Gary Havel Jr. and I started our *21-day Hugging Journey on Loving Yourself in the Now*, we proclaimed it to the world live on Facebook, and then used each other to provide support, accountability, and direction. We started off our journey by taking our shirts off on Facebook Live, both literally and figuratively. At the time, Gary had already lost over forty pounds from an earlier journey, and I was inspired by his idea to show our "soft underbellies" to the world. When we did that live on video, he weighed about 295 pounds and he said to me, "Stone, as much as I love Buddha, I don't want to look like him anymore." There we were live with our shirts off and our love handles hanging out for the world to see. Both of us exposed from the waist up. Now, I am not advocating for you to take your clothes off, but I talk with my clients all the time about being vulnerable and loving ourselves exactly as we are. This is the starting place for creating meaningful change.

Gary noted that he didn't complete a prior fitness hugging journey, and he explained that he stopped on day 15 and "it kind of felt like a failure." He explained, "I missed one day, and I felt like I could never get back on track and I just got too busy, and in my own head, and by 15 days, it wasn't going as powerfully as I hoped, and I guess I just gave up." We discussed how he had some of these feelings on other days, and yet didn't stop. The challenge is to create a structure that supports you even when it gets most difficult. In addition, missing one day, although not ideal, is not something to beat oneself up about. It's a learning moment, and the hugging ambassador has gone on to complete many hugging journeys, giving out thousands of hugs, hundreds of 21-second hugs, and inspiring countless huggers.

On his next 21-Day Hugging Journey for "Fitness and Being Fully Present Now" he made a commitment to practice yoga every day of his hugging journey. He signed up for a yoga studio special that he found, "Thirty dollars for unlimited yoga for thirty days." During this hugging journey, he did yoga almost every day, and many days, twice. He found yoga to be extremely grounding, and to be a natural fit with mindful hugging. Approximately a week into his journey, he powerfully encouraged me to join the studio as well, and we did a half dozen yoga classes together. This deepened our commitment to each other, to our health, and it helped connect us more deeply with our bodies. He wanted me to remind readers, "even if you don't feel like doing it, do it, because I feel so much better after I do it, and I often really don't want to, especially some of those days I did yoga twice, and my body was pretty sore from hiking a couple of miles."

One of the instructors, Joe, had a deep impact on how I view yoga that I want to share. I think it also provides insight into how to think about your 21-Day Hugging Journey. He explained how each of the poses we did during his class were suggestions, and that a true yogi listens to his/her body. He gave the straightforward and essential advice, "listen to your body, and if it hurts don't do it. There is no magical pose that I can push you into that will make you reach enlightenment; listen to your body and do what feels good. Pay attention to your breathing and see yourself from outside yourself."

This underscored and solidified everything that I know from past yoga classes and hugging. In this moment right now, take stock of your body. Notice how it feels. If you want, close your eyes and do a body scan. Notice where you are holding pressure. See your feet in your mind's eye. Are you wearing socks? How do the socks feel against your skin? Are they warm or cold? Simply notice. Are you outside? Can you feel the sun on your body? Are you inside? Is it cool? Is the air-conditioning on? Are you cold? Slow down and notice your body as if you were standing outside of yourself, looking at you. Notice what you look like, without judging. Simply notice how you are sitting, if you are leaning forward or back. See yourself in this moment. Really look. If you are a thirty-nine-year-old woman or a sixty-seven-year-old man, really look at yourself. Get in touch with yourself and with your body. Now, from this place, start to accept whatever it is you see. Even begin to embrace it all, the challenges this person you are looking at has had. Really look and let this wash over you in whatever point you are in your life. Noticing and not judging. If you start to judge, notice that you are doing that, and then come back to really seeing yourself and your physicality. Can you see different parts of your body with your eyes closed? This all fits in with your fitness, being able to see everything about who you are, accepting yourself in this moment, and at the same time, having a commitment to your health.

Yoga is one highly effective tool to help you increase your self-awareness and peace of mind. You can start to see that it fits fluidly with a 21-Day Hugging Journey. Likely there are many yoga studios around you, and perhaps you are already engaging in yoga once a week, or a few times a week. If you are in a more remote area, or you find the classes are too expensive, you can also find great free classes on YouTube. You can use your 21-Day Hugging Journey to try it for the first time, or to deepen your yoga practice or other routines that ground you. Allow this self-embrace to empower and support you in what really matters to you the most. Move in that direction in a loving way for 21 days.

Skip to Your Lou Today

As small children, some of us skipped about with freedom and ease, and that's an awesome thing. Too often, we lose touch with our playful side. Whether or not you can remember skipping as a child, now is the time to experience it anew, or reconnect with that inner you. Whether it's actually skipping, or another behavior, let your inner child come out and play. Give yourself the hug of skipping through life, today, now. If you feel confused about what to do, start by literally skipping around your house. I just got up and did some skipping myself with a dear "stranger," who I met on a 21-Day Hugging Journey, and became friends with; her name is Kathy Lee James. I was at her house, working on *Hug Therapy*, and getting her valuable feedback. I was sharing about this section with her , and decided to skip around her house to feel the experience more than just think about it.

There is a useful lesson here. It's one thing to be up in our heads, and another to be in action. When we take action, we create possibilities and we don't exactly know what will happen next. This can be scary, as well as fun and exciting. When I skipped around her house, I woke her bulldog, Franklin, sleeping nearby. He was apparently quite pleased with my sudden energetic movements, to the point that Franklin began to "hug" my leg. This is something that definitely would not have happened if I hadn't started to skip. The reality is that it gave us both a lot of laughter, and it was my first "hug from a bulldog." The point is, each little tweak or change we make in our actions opens up a whole new realm. I will also skip today outside of the home, and see what is created. Understand that literally skipping is an excellent concrete launching pad, and that anything that has the fun and playful feel of skipping can fit beautifully into your hugging journey.

The more I skip, the more I notice that it adds a feeling of lightness and playfulness I don't experience when I simply walk somewhere. It almost has a quality of floating or briefly flying. Will you skip today? Perhaps a little bit right now at your house, or wherever you are reading this? If you won't, or are reluctant to skip, take a moment to notice what comes up for you, and get in touch with what is holding you back. It's not right or wrong to skip, and I want you to consider exploring what takes you out of your comfort zone a bit and allows you the freedom to explore new and life affirming movement. If skipping isn't for you, or isn't for you right now or today, then what can you choose to do that takes you a bit out of your comfort zone and puts you in the "hugging zone," leaving you with a sense of creativity, growth, exploration, or triumph?

Don't Make Your Bed or Choose to Make Your Bed Right Now

Our happiness and satisfaction in our life's work all comes down to awareness about each moment. Any tool that can increase our understanding of what causes us to tune out and/or go on automatic pilot is valuable. Helping us to better

Hug Therapy

be able to accept and ultimately love ourselves, and make educated choices about how to spend our precious present moments. That is why I *love* the hug so much. It forces us (if we choose to hug or be aware of the space of a hug) to be fully present. Another way to be fully aware is to choose to do something the opposite way of how we generally choose to do it.

For example, which hand do you brush your teeth with every night? If you aren't brushing your teeth every night, I strongly encourage you to start. I think by including that in the book that my dentist will want to give me a longer hug! Seriously though, which hand do you use? I will assume that you are a righty, since Google says that 90 percent of people are right-handed. Tonight, I want you to brush your teeth with your opposite or non-dominant hand. I am going to do it right now, so that I can write this part as descriptively as possible. Just a minute. Look at me killing two birds with one stone, brushing my teeth at 11:56 a.m. on a Friday and delving deeper into the present. If you want, and you have access to your toothbrush, do the exercise of brushing with the hand you don't usually use, see what you notice and then we can compare notes. If you don't have access to your toothbrush right now, I will tell you about my experience and then you can give it a go tonight or in the morning.

The first thing I noticed is that I wanted to choke up on the toothbrush and hold it closer to the top, because it was a bit harder for me to control. It was almost as if someone else was brushing my teeth, just a little. Something that I do more or less in my sleep with my right hand, with my left, it took some real focus. In fact, when I wanted to turn the toothbrush around in my mouth, not only did I have a bit of a hard time, but at one point I felt like I might drop it completely. I don't think I was actually that close, but for a moment it felt like I might.

The point of this exercise is to be increasingly aware of how often we are in a space of acting automatically without awareness. Remember, when this is the case, it's as if we are literally losing moments of life we can never get back. Driving is one example where we often can pass twenty minutes, and have no recollection of what happened or what we did. Think how rich of an opportunity it is to recapture these moments in a way that we are actively experiencing them. For example, noticing each time that we see the color blue on our drive, or how many shades of blue we can notice. How does this relate to your 21-Day Hugging Journey? Being fully present in this moment is a huge hug, and gives you the flexibility to choose how you spend your time. We often hear people speaking about how valuable time is and how limited it is, and the more we can be fully engaged in our time, the more we can squeeze out of it, and appreciate the richness of life. The difference, in short, might be two different ways of drinking a glass of freshly squeezed orange juice. With the first, it could be we are just drinking and thinking about the meeting we will have later in the day, but with the second, we are really tasting it, feeling the texture, feeling the sweetness and depth of juice fresh from the orange. Any exercises you can do to increase your experience of being fully present in *this* moment is worthwhile, and some might even say hug-worthy. Hug that juice!

Another exercise that often impacts us is whether you generally make your bed each morning or not. Keep in mind there is no judgment about whether you do or don't make your bed. Again, it's about being present.

Notice what you usually do around making your bed, or not, and then choose to do the opposite either today or tomorrow. By breaking your routine, you will notice some things, and thus begins the discovery process. It's not right or wrong to make your bed or not to make it. Notice what it means to you when you make it or when you don't, and how this leaves you feeling about yourself. Give yourself freedom to play and explore. Some huggers have told me that spending time to truly make the bed with intensity and focus can be a Zen experience. What can you discover in this act or any other act in which you might be caught in routine?

Often our routines leave us out of touch. I find, for myself, it can be an awesome embrace to slow down and appreciate that changing the kitty litter, for example, can be soothing, and helps me appreciate why I choose to engage in this activity, and how it is essential in the fabric of my life. It can be an expression of loving my cat, and what having a pet means to our family. The alternative is that I can deeply resent the kitty litter changing, and lose those minutes forever by going through the motions. If this is the case about how we are operating in any part of our lives, then we really need to take a deeper look, and determine if a pet is the right fit for our family.

The Adventurous Hug

Do something daring, something a bit risky, that makes you feel alive and stimulates you. It could be walking around the house naked, or playing your music really loud and dancing your heart out. Maybe throw an all by yourself dance party. What awakens your sense of adventure? This is about you literally and figuratively taking your shirt off and allowing your soft underbelly to feel the breeze or the warmth of the sun on your skin. What can you say or do in this moment that reminds you that you are alive, and lets you share with the world your love of life and the people around you?

It can be something in the more immediate moment or taking the leap to do something you have always wanted to do, but have been holding back. Perhaps you have always wanted to ride in a hot air balloon or drive the California coastline in a convertible.

An example of this in my life was taking the hugging movement to Cuba. It was a spontaneous trip, the timing came together, and it felt right, so I embraced it. I didn't know what to expect, or exactly how it would turn out. It was a big financial investment, and I really didn't know how the Cuban people would respond to the idea of longer hugs and "the space of a hug." I had a translator, but a lot can still get lost in translation. This was the first country outside the US that I brought hugging to, and I am excited about exploring other countries and cultures to learn how they understand and experience hugs so we can learn from each other.

In Cuba, it was also very cool, because I had the opportunity to work with a professional film crew to capture some of this adventure. Some highlights of my trip included having a hug with Cuba's Olympic boxing coach, and seeing him training Olympic athletes, one of whom later went on to win the gold. While I was there, I hugged countless people from all over the world, and became very close to some outstanding people. This was the trip of a lifetime, and it was one of my most adventurous and rewarding self-hugs. The Cuban people were amazing. I worked on the language barrier with guides and interpreters, and learned that *abrazo* is "hugging" in Spanish, as well as many other nuances about this amazing culture.

Yoga in the Plane

This example is something I have done, and I will talk about the specifics and what it meant and still means to me; this is designed to get you thinking outside of the box about how you can creatively and spontaneously love yourself.

On plane flights sometimes, it can be a good idea to get up and walk a bit, to allow for some stretching and to help with lower back issues that many people experience. For years I have been doing yoga, but never felt that I could really do it on the plane, because there isn't space, or at least so I thought. One day when my back was feeling sore and the flight felt particularly long, I had a "hug-storm." I could do yoga in the aisle of the plane. Or could I? At first, I was hesitant, what would others think? It was/is a pretty tight space, and I didn't want to upset anyone. Would the stewards and stewardesses even allow it? Then I went for it, and it was cool. I may have gotten some strange looks, but no one really seemed to care. I was in downward dog, flying on the way to my destination, able to stretch my body in a way that felt amazing, I felt really good to me and my back, and I totally felt alive in that moment. These are the little moments that are so critical, this is what I want you to uncover on your journey. And as you do, share your insights and discoveries with others, to enrich and nurture their lives as well.

Consider the things that you would like to do sometimes and hold back. Nothing dangerous or illegal, but what can you do to have more fun and love yourself? Another example tied into airports is that on a very long layover, I took my shoes off and was gliding through the airport in my socks, like I was cross-country skiing. My music was on, and I had an amazing time during a period when I might otherwise have been bored and frustrated that my plane kept being delayed. I definitely got some funny looks and many smiles, thumbs up, and encouragement. We have all heard it before, and I think it is worth repeating, "Life is short."

Now you may be reading some of these things and thinking, this guy is a bit off the deep end: hugging strangers, yoga on the plane, gliding around the airport in his socks. You might be right. Certainly off the deep end of hugging myself and the world. Keep in mind these are examples from my life to illustrate how you might embrace yourself. I need for you to look deeply at your own comfort zone and what might enrich and nurture you. You don't need to slide around the airport in your socks, but if you want to…

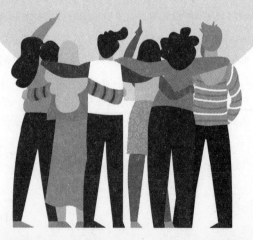

Part IV

Embrace Life

The following are exercises designed to give you an example of how to embrace life more fully. What is the deep end of life? What does it mean to dive into it from a hugging standpoint? The first step is to complete a radically transparent inventory of what you have created so far, and what you still want to create. It's looking at life from a different angle. If you knew, for example, that you only had a year to live, how happy would you be with what you have achieved? How would you shift your focus to dive deeper? The 21-Day Hugging Journey gives you a chance to do this introspection, and then have accountability to yourself, and to a hugging accountability buddy to make it happen. Here are a few examples of diving deeper into life.

Go See a Movie with You

Sometimes, we hold off on doing things that we really want to do or see, because we don't want to be alone. Doing activities with friends, family, or a romantic partner can be rewarding, meaningful, and fun. Choosing to do something alone or, more accurately, with yourself, is an essential component of embracing life. Too many times, people will not attend an event that they want, whether it's a lecture, concert, movie, or dance, simply because they are uncomfortable going alone. Trust that choosing to go by yourself and have you be enough is a huge step to diving deeper into life. It can be great to have a friend or a date with you for an event, but it can be great to go with yourself.

Let yourself have the full experience of being with you. Notice the survival mechanism kicking in, trying to tell you that there is something wrong. Notice that voice, and how powerful it is not to listen to it. Instead, embrace a solo activity. Notice how the voice gets more agitated when others are at the movie with a group of friends, family, or on a date. Perhaps it might say, "what's wrong with you that you are here alone." Notice this voice and how it attempts to manipulate you and make you feel 'less than.' Notice how much you can enjoy being with you, and be secure in the reality that you don't need anyone else and are brave to go after what you want. Let yourself have all the thoughts and feelings that come along for the ride.

It's not the primary intention of this exercise, but notice how often you are surprised as you meet new friends, romantic interests, etc. when you go somewhere with yourself. You are more likely to connect with others when you are doing an activity that you enjoy and are in your own zone, because you are pursuing something that you genuinely love or care about. The intention isn't to meet anyone else, but this is more likely when you are in a space in which you are loving yourself and engaging in activities you truly enjoy.

Donate for Seven Days in a Row

What causes matter to you the most? Start to think about where and how you want to spend your money. The amount you choose is less significant than the fact that you take action, starting today. Pick seven of the causes that matter the most to you, and figure out why and how you want to give the donation. You may also choose to donate your time. There are so many philanthropic organizations working day in and day out to support causes you believe in passionately. Notice, if you support one today, in the space of a hug, how much better you feel about the world in which you live. We often think about or consider these types of charitable hugs, but your challenge is to take the action today. Thinking about giving someone a hug, and actually giving them a hug are very different. Just as considering the hug of giving your time or money to a charitable organization, and actually doing it are distinct.

Regardless of the sum of money, place your focus on the power of being in action. Discover how it feels to give for seven consecutive days in a row to causes that matter to you deeply. Pay attention to the impact this has on you when you incorporate giving into your day for seven days in a row. If you let it, this hug can inspire the rest of your day, remind you of who you are, and what really matters. Do not think of this as an exercise in your head; think of it as a consistent impact that you choose to have in the world.

Do Something Bold and Perhaps Scary

First, what scares you? To what do you say, "I will never do that"? Why? Is it public speaking? We know that this is one of the biggest fears for people. The point is not for you to become a public speaker, unless that is what you really want. The objective is to identify and have clarity about what you fear. The goal is to be radically transparent with yourself about something that you feel is missing and that frightens you. Perhaps, you never learned to swim, maybe you have a fear of heights, maybe you are shy in some situations in which you really want to be bold? The first key is to take a hard look at what scares you. For some, the last exercise of seeing a movie alone may have been one of those fears.

These fears, or reluctance to overcome certain obstacles in our lives can hold us back in much bigger ways. When we know ourselves to be someone who can't handle small setbacks, it has the potential to leave us questioning ourselves in other domains.

Identify what that fear is and pick something concrete that you can do today to overcome it. For example, if public speaking is a fear that you believe is holding you back, join a club today, such as Toastmasters, to allow yourself the opportunity to learn about public speaking, and how to deal effectively with fear. First, be radically transparent with yourself and identify this is a fear that you are tackling. Then, start to express your intent to those around you, because your words are powerful. By setting the ball in motion and committing to taking the first step, you create a world of possibility. Even as you are scheduling or attending the first meeting, yes, you may feel anxious, and that's okay. Give that anxiety a hug. Because you are in action, and the anxiety will come and go. You are vitally alive and in the process of embracing one of your fears, and creating a life which you are charged about.

By this point, you are probably pretty clear that I think hugs and hugging are potent and valuable on many levels. To underscore this point, I want to share something that has taken me out of my comfort zone. Remember, this is an example of something that clicks for me, and I encourage you to find something catered to your own needs, and not necessarily what I did.

You may have seen a preview of what I'm referring to on my website or in one of the videos online. It has been very meaningful to me at different times to have HUG shaved in the back of my head. First, I love to have a somewhat subliminal message on my head that lets people know wherever I go what I think is important. It is my hope that people who read it are amused and/or feel more likely to connect in a positive way with people around them. It has also resulted in many people approaching me, wanting to know more about why I do it, and what a 21-Day Hugging Journey is. It has also created many awesome conversations and connections.

I have also let children use markers to color in the HUG on my head, as this is a fun activity that allows their expression to brighten the world wherever I go. The process of having HUG sheared into my head has gone through many iterations, and I have enjoyed the journey. I am not sure what will be next—and that's half the fun. The point is, sometimes I feel shy about having HUG on my head. Perhaps it works better in some settings than in others. People likely have all kinds of different ideas when they see me. I like to think that among other things, I am a walking billboard for world peace. What do you want to do that is a bit weird, distinct, or magical that will light up your day and possibly have a meaningful impact on the world?

Fitness, Fun, and Raising Awareness

Train for a 5k run and get friends and family involved, making it a combo of fitness, fun, and raising awareness for a cause that really matters to you!

Fitness is something that everyone consistently bumps up against in life, as we discussed in the self-hug section. Whether we have a regular routine or not, we can't help but be aware to varying degrees of how much fitness impacts our health, mood, and longevity. You can't turn on the TV or the internet for more than a minute without being assaulted by the newest get trim program, diet pills, or beauty/health advertisements.

This life hug throws you into a healthy fitness program of your own design with friends and family. You have all the freedom to create and make it work in a way that works best for you. Choose a 5K or longer race, depending on your current level of fitness, that supports a charity that you believe in.

Then reach out to your friends and family about why you are supporting this charity, and get them excited about joining you. Explain how you want to train together as a group for a period of time that feels right prior to the event. Get a list of the different people you want on the team, and have fun creating a team name, and anything else that enhances the process. Be silly, be creative, and think outside the box. Give lots of hugs as well.

Pair each person on your team with a 5K hugging training buddy to help them workout three to four times a week (look at tools online such as Couch to 5K which give concrete training steps) and build up to a level of exercise that increases each person's fitness. It doesn't matter if people are walking, jogging, or running the 5K. Being a part of a shared goal, working together as a team toward fitness, and supporting a charitable cause is an awesome hug on many levels.

Multiple 21-Second Hugs Today

Okay, awesome. You are this far into learning about the power of hugging, going on 21-Day Hugging Journey's and 21-second hugs. Have you had a 21-second hug yet? Mind you, 21-seconds is a pretty looooooong time for those of us used to standard hugging. In fact, go back to the beginning of this paragraph and read up until about *here*—that is 21-seconds. Who can you hug for this long?

Initially, people think that it needs to be someone they are very close to, and that is a great place to start. The question is: have you broached having a 21-second hug with those people to who you are closest? If not, why not? You certainly don't have to, not by any means. As has been discussed previously, 21-second hugs release oxytocin, and are good for your stress response, immune systems, and blood pressure, as well as benefitting the person who is lucky enough to be hugging you.

To be clear, the idea goes even beyond the 21 seconds to getting "lost in the hug." The objective is to let yourself experience the hug as meditative. In other words, you are taking some deep breaths and not worrying about the time at all, allowing yourself to deeply connect with this other person. During many of my longer and more powerful hugs, I have not only lost track of time, I have also felt that I have a profound connection with this other human, and an awareness that we are made of the same stuff. I once heard that we are all simply stardust, and during a long, healing, and deeply connected hug it starts to feel like that to me.

Once you are clear you want to have a 21-second hug, and you have another individual, who is also clear they want to share a 21-second hug with you, follow my coaching instructions:

Step One: Make sure you are both comfortable based on size and how you are hugging. For example, have your bodies comfortably fitting together. We don't want anyone standing on their tip-toes or bending way down to where it will be uncomfortable or put strain on their back. That would only work for a few seconds, and the goal is a hug that lasts a minimum of 21 seconds. If one person is much taller, it may be helpful for the other to stand on a bench or stair so that it is comfortable for both.

Step Two: each of you take a few deep breaths, as if you are meditating—in through the nose and out through the mouth. Don't worry about how many, just breathe deeply. As you do this more, you will notice that your bodies start to regulate with each other.

Step Three: (maybe this should be Step One—you will get the idea), be radically transparent with each other during the hug. It's okay to talk some. This is a balance. You don't want to talk so much that you take away from the power and meditative qualities of the hug, you do want to express yourself. So, if for any reason you want the hug to stop before 21-seconds, definitely express that, and stop hugging. This is not a roller coaster where once you get in, you are locked in for the ride. This is totally up to you and there is nothing right or wrong about stopping at five seconds or going to thirty-five seconds. This is all about your comfort level with each other and how long you each choose to hug.

Sometimes, when I am having a longer hug, and it's in public, I will notice that I am talking a bit to the other hugger about how it feels to be having such a long hug in a public place. We just notice together how this feels, and the way that it seems to transform the entire space we are in. Why are they hugging for that long? What's going on? Who is that guy? Does he have hug shaved into his hair? The point is, we are having an impact on the space around us, and it is okay to talk with each other about whatever we want in the literal space of a hug. Other times, it is common for people to say things like "I really needed that" or "Wow, this isn't like any other hug I have ever had. I feel so peaceful," or "I can see how this works and it's so hard for me to really let myself relax." This will be distinct for each 21-second hug. The dynamics of the two people who are coming together, their hugging history, their upbringing around touch—if they have ever been abused, are introverted or extroverted—all of this will have an impact on some level. And if they have chosen to have a long hug (and get lost in the hug), all of this will start to wash away as the oxytocin washes over the two of you.

The Final Step: The way I like to end hugs, and particularly long hugs that I have gotten lost in, is to leave the person you have just hugged with "the hug of your words." Tell them what you really want them to know. Tell them how much they mean to you, and how they inspire or ground you. Share with them what really matters, what you would want them to know at the core. Sometimes, it helps to imagine you might never see them again (which sadly, powerfully, and existentially is always a real possibility). I will often say at the end of a hug, although I vary it based on the person, the moment, and what feels right and most meaningful, "this hug will leave you with lightness and joy and a profound sense of who you are in the world."

The other thing that I am fond of saying at the end of a hug is "hugging powers activate!" I say this, because I believe that we have both been charged with powerful and positive hugging energy, leaving us each with a good and healthy charge. Some of the things that may have been weighing on us have likely been lightened, and the combination of the oxytocin and experiencing the good in humanity leaves me feeling more ready and able to deal powerfully with whatever comes next. I believe as more and more of us are continually activating our hugging powers, we will begin to see more and more beautiful things happening in the world.

So again, I ask you, have you had a 21-second hug yet? Because this exercise involves having a bunch of them today—if you choose to take it on. And I have news for you: you can have a 21-second hug or longer with a stranger, if you both want to hug, and clearly communicate this to one another. I have had this rich experience many times, and it is empowering, uplifting, and has left me feeling alive and radiant. "Stranger" is a word that we use for someone that we don't know, and yet, what moves someone from being a stranger to a dear friend? By engaging in a discussion about the power of hugging, and having a hug or a 21-second hug, you can actively answer this question in your life. Now, get out there and hug. Let us know on social media, or however you would like to share, about your 21-second hugs, and how they impact you and those around you. I am happy to answer any questions you have before you experience the unique beauty of getting "lost in a hug." This is when you plan to have a 21-second hug, and you have such a lovely experience that no one is keeping track of time, and you imagine it might have been a minute or more. Time is a funny thing, and getting "lost in a hug" with a close friend, family member or anyone you trust/care about can be a brilliant life moment—or many moments!

Radically Tell the World about Your Hugging Experience

Okay, by this point you have likely seen some miraculous stuff happen for you, and those around you, based on your loving choices and the power of hugging. How can you most effectively share this in the world? There is a lot of pain and suffering out there that we are bombarded with on the news. Whether it is the most recent mass shooting or the natural disasters like the one in Puerto Rico. Consider, that you are holding the antidote to this suffering in your hands. You have something powerful that can spread love and connection in the world. How can you most effectively share this hugging technology with other people and continue to allow your love and affinity for your friends, family, country, and the world to grow? There are hundreds of different ways and each person reading the book will have their own creative path. As the Hug Doctor, it is my goal to support and empower each and every one of you. Hugging technology offers foundational tools to help us move toward a more peaceful world—one hug at a time. What powerful hug steps will you take today?

Share Your Romantic Feelings

If you are single tell someone whom you have passionate feelings for or a crush on how you truly feel. Why have you been holding back? Their reply isn't the focus. You embrace life when you step out of your comfort zone and radically transparently tell someone how you feel. Love like this. Although it takes a leap. It makes life simpler, more joyful, and pure. You may be tickled by what you discover regardless of their response.

Consider that you have nothing to lose, and everything to gain. They don't reciprocate, that's okay, give the feelings that come up a hug. Are there tears? Let them flow. By holding on to the fantasy of them liking you, it was the anti-hug. It was getting in the way of a reality that really works for you. Now, you can grieve and move powerfully forward, connecting with someone else that does reciprocate your feelings. Life is short, and as my grandmother said, "there is a lid for every pot." Don't get caught focusing your energy, heart, and love on someone who isn't interested. They might not be interested due to bunches of reasons that have nothing to do with you. If they aren't right, they aren't right. Although you were radically transparent with them, and now, because that kind of self-expression is powerful, it may create other opportunities. It's fueled by confidence, and a belief that you and your love matter. The point is *express your love and feelings.* Take the leap. No matter what happens, this is positive movement forward at hugging yourself and creating a reality you love.

Part V

Embrace Others

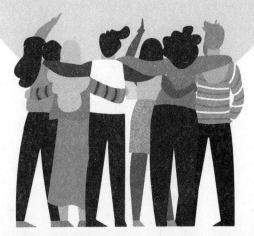

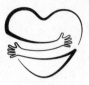

Hug with Consent or Not at All

The mission of *Hug Therapy* is to create connection through physical, virtual, or metaphorical hugs. A hug can be an embrace, a kind thought, or an inspiration. It can create closeness or synergy. It is never intended to make anyone feel claustrophobic, constrained, or uncomfortable. It is the hugger's responsibility to be respectful of the huggee. In other words, meet them at their comfort level. Some people may not like hugs that involve physical touch. Respect that. Trust that they know exactly what works for them; don't ever push or pressure. Let them know that if they want a physical hug, it is there for the asking. In the meantime, bathe them in the space of hugging by being warm and accepting, which requires no physical contact.

Some people may not be open to physical hugs, perhaps because of something that happened in the past. Or they may simply prefer not to be touched, or not to be touched by you. To be insensitive to their reluctance to be hugged is exactly the opposite of what *Hug Therapy* is all about.

When you ask someone, "Would you like a hug?" or "Would you like a twenty-one-second hug?" if you don't receive an enthusiastic YES, don't do it. This is not an urgent matter. Nobody needs a hug. It can be beneficial, desirable, or fun, but it is not something to be rushed or pushed. Trust that you are the space of a hug by waiting. If your instincts are telling you NO, or not right now, trust them. Again, remember that hugging doesn't always involve a physical embrace. It may be more important to create a warm and accepting space.

Being with others, looking into their eyes, listening to them—all of that can be considered a hug. Letting them know that they are loved deeply for who they really are is the hug we are after. If one day they want a physical hug, that's great. If one day they feel safe and trusting enough to have that connection, that's wonderful. But it isn't necessary. That moment might be today, it might be in five years, or it might be never. The space of hugging doesn't require any physical contact.

All of this takes a deep level of communication. It takes really paying attention, caring, and investing in the connection between you and each person you encounter. People will be everywhere on the openness-to-physical-contact continuum. It is important to communicate with them about where they are and what works best for them.

If someone has given 100 percent consent to being hugged, and even enthusiastically agreed to a 21-second hug, you can say "just say when" to let them know it's okay to stop whenever they choose. If the first hug is twelve seconds, that's okay. If it's seven seconds, that's okay, too. The number of seconds is not the point. In fact, it can often be a distraction. The idea is to relax into the hug and be present and connected to the other person.

What you want is an extended hug that may release oxytocin. Don't count. If the other person wants to stop, *stop*. This will build trust and comfort, and aid in nurturing the connection. Next time, they may want a longer hug. Let each individual decide. Any clear, consensual communication between two people leads to a positive outcome—a model for connecting in the world and all that can result from such connection.

WHY THIS MATTERS

This is a playbook from which to create healthy relationships in any situation—a way to be in the space of a hug (loving and accepting), regardless of the situation.

ACTION

Think about the people in your life you feel closest to. How will you decide how long you want a hug to last? How much does it have to do with your history with them? How much does it have to do with how you feel around them? How much do you trust this person? Who initiates hugs? How do you treat them, and what do they mean to you?

The following are seven exercises to give you a powerful sample of what it means to embrace everyone around you.

Tell Those Who Raised You What They Really Mean to You

Tell your parents, or those who raised you, that you love them, and really let them feel your love. Tell them as though this is the last time that you will ever be able to share with them. Whether they are alive or dead, straight from your heart, radically and transparently, share with them the impact they have had on you. If they are alive, tell them in person, if possible. Regardless, let this conversation leave you feeling complete, knowing that you have shared with them what deeply matters to you and what you think it is imperative for them to know. Imagine this is your very last chance to "hug them with your words."

If they are deceased, say it out loud to them. Record it on your phone, or put it in a written letter. Whatever mode of communication seems most powerful for you to express what they mean to you, use it. Even if they are gone, what they mean to you is still valid and real. Whether the relationship was a challenging/complicated one, or a solid and straightforward one, it is time to become complete with what was, and embrace the role that they had in your life. It may not have been exactly what you wanted, but consider that it is in the past, and this is the foundation that you have moving forward, and it impacts all your current relationships.

Give Your 21-Day Hugging Accountability Buddy a Big Hug

Reach out and give your 21-day hugging accountability buddy the biggest hug. What can you do to surprise and delight them and acknowledge them for what they've accomplished in the world? Let them know how they inspire you. Let your love shine through in this hug. Show them how special they are to you. Perhaps write them a poem or bake them a cake. What can you do that will give them a powerful surge moving forward?

Hug a Stranger

Be fully present to the people around you. Really see them. Be in the space of a hug and be supportive of others. Breathe, slow down, connect, and be with the people around you. Start to understand more deeply that we are all profoundly connected, and that *there really are no strangers*. Consider offering a hug to a stranger if it feels right.

Hug It Forward

What does this mean? It means a million things. It means holding the door open; it means smiling; it means not snapping at somebody when "they deserve it." It means seeing that something needs to change, seeing how change will impact others, and making this change happen. It means not living a selfish life. It means embracing "there but for the grace of God go I." It means opening your heart. It means not beating yourself up when your heart doesn't feel open. It means hugging more. It means breathing more. It means telling others what they really mean to you. It means slowing down. It means loving yourself deeply enough to get caught up in the magic of who you are, and how you can powerfully impact the world around you.

Shower Friends and Family with Sweet Notes

Sometimes, arguably often, it is the little things that make the most difference. We have each heard this concept before, and we know that there is some truth to it. This hug is about taking action in this arena. Who can you express your love to, with some little notes of affection? Someone that you haven't taken the time to hug due to being caught up in the "rat race" or "hustle and bustle of life?" What would it be like to leave your spouse a little note on the pillow this morning or put one in your kid's lunch pail? This doesn't have to take a ton of time, energy, or money. It's allowing yourself the freedom to play and discover what you can do with a little note, flower, or other gesture that will touch you both. You can't give a hug without getting one in return.

Set Up a 21-Second Hug Zone

Now you have experienced for yourself the power of the 21-second hug and you have gotten lost in some hugs. How about creating a zone in which people can choose to enter if they would like a 21-second hug? What a fun way to spend an afternoon or a few hours on a weekday!

Creatively make this a zone where people know that you are willing and want to give them a long hug. Teach others about the power of hugging. Create a profound space in which people can learn more about the different components of a hug, and more specifically, what the hug has meant for you. If you are reading this and thinking, well, for me it would be more about creating something at my kid's school that provides tutoring for an hour after school or some other kind of outreach, then this is your 21-second hug zone. It doesn't have to involve 21-seconds of physical connection, but it can—whatever you choose to create.

Allow this exercise to give you the freedom to create and explore a space where you see a need, and have a desire to fulfill. This may occur solo or you may provide the resources of friends, family, or finances to put your plan in action. Consider what you really want to see in your community, and what you would feel proud of being a part of at the end of the day. So often, our focus gets fixated on our own survival, our retirement, or next vacation that we lose sight of something in our own backyard that makes a world of difference for us and those around us. That is the power of hugging. Again, you can't give one without getting one.

Perhaps you are reading this and thinking, well, I am already part of the PTA or volunteer at the soup kitchen. Awesome. Now how can you supercharge this activity, so that it is most meaningful for you and those around you. This kind of work takes a village to stay motivated and effective. Too often, we do something as a routine and start to lose track of our initial passion. How can you tweak, change, or enhance your "21 Second Hug Zone" to allow increased vitality for you and for those whom you want to impact?

Life Prolonging Hugs

When you connect with people in your community and immediate surroundings, research suggests that you are not only extending the quality of your life in the moment, but also your longevity. Blue Zones, seven locations in the world where people are living past hundred years, have been studied extensively. (One such place is Sardinia in the Mediterranean.) The findings suggest that more face-to-face contact and physical contact, such as hugging, has "stunning impacts" for our health. Look for Susan Pinker's TED Talk entitled, "The secret to living longer may be your social life," easily available online. In it, she describes her research, the importance of living in a village, and how "building it and sustaining it is a matter of life and death."

Part VI

Summing Up and Moving Forward

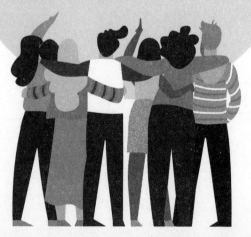

The Journey Begins—#21DAYHUG

"And those who were seen dancing were thought to be insane by
those who could not hear the music."

—Friedrich Nietzsche

Now that you have a better understanding of all the tools
at your disposal for a 21-day hugging journey, you can
appreciate it's a concrete yet amazingly adaptable structure
for hearing the musical soundtrack of your life. Consider that
it's always playing, but that as humans, we get so caught up
in the struggle and buzz of anxiety, we drown out our own
beautiful, one-of-a-kind, inspiring soundtrack. Start to slow
down, tune in, and listen deeply. Listen closely—can you hear
your music? It is always playing. When you begin to hear it,
let it wash over you in a way that nurtures, empowers, and
delights you. Your power often gets buried under self-talk,
stress, and pressure. This journey will give you the power,
within the space of a hug, to clearly identify what is holding

you back—giving you the freedom to reconnect with what matters to you, and to live an increasingly inspired life.

To this end, I invite you on the journey. This is not the kind of journey where you start out in one place and end up somewhere different. This journey is about being just where you are—completely present in your life right now. It's about silencing all the self-talk, should haves, and to-do lists in your mind long enough to hug someone who matters to you.

This journey will be distinct for each person who takes it on. My assurance to you is that, wherever your travels take you, you are embarking on a journey of discovery, value, and love. The beauty of the hugging journey is that it meets you exactly where you are, and opens that next window of growth and connection. These are to be twenty-one days in which you allow hugging to be the framework from which to see the world. This can unfold in a multitude of ways. The objective is to view your world in a way in which you identify your power and act on it. The journey may involve physical hugging, virtual hugging, and/or the space of a hug.

If you want to take action, pick someone you care about, and give that person a big hug—not a quick squeeze of greeting or affection, but a hug that is distinct from any you have given to this point, and is a line in the sand about the journey you are going on; a hug that requires a warning beforehand, and a discussion afterward. A hug that communicates with crystal clarity, "You, fellow human, make my world larger, richer, and more brilliant." Then, tomorrow, and the day after, and the day after that, repeat the process with other people you love, until you have hugged—really hugged—twenty-one people.

Chances are you have never hugged anyone or been hugged for twenty-one seconds. It's not an everyday occurrence, but together we can make it one. Hugs are wonderful. They feel good. They transmit all kinds of positive energy. But twenty-one-second hugs are also powerful. There is no way to describe them; they require actual experience to be understood. This is not an intellectual exercise.

It takes a while to form a new habit. I promise you that by the end of twenty-one days, you will be hooked on the hugging habit. But just to be sure, before you take the first step on this journey, make a commitment to sticking with it for twenty-one days. Tell someone, tweet it to your followers, announce it on Facebook, or blog about it. When you make a promise in such a public forum, you are much more likely to keep it.

One of the most powerful ways to go on the hugging journey was blazed by hugging ambassador Gary Havel Jr. This is to take the journey on Facebook Live (you can see his journey by searching for "Gary Havel Jr. Gary Day #1" on YouTube).

The beauty of this way of completing this journey is that it connects the world with you, and gives each individual going on the journey a rich platform from which to spread the power of hugging. By being radically transparent with Facebook (or whatever live social media you wish to use), you're allowing connections to be created and possibilities to blossom.

Even if you are already a comfortable hugger, the first few days may feel a bit awkward. Like any new undertaking, it may take a while to get in the rhythm, and then you'll wonder how you ever lived without your daily twenty-one-second hug.

If you're thinking, "Okay, the whole idea sounds like fun, but why am I committing to do this for twenty-one days?" That's a great question—and only you can answer it. It will give you a platform to step out of automatic mode and be alive in the world. It can deepen and enhance your connection to those with whom you are already super close. There is nothing automatic about a long, heartfelt hug. You must be fully present to give or receive one.

The physical hug is mind-blowingly powerful, and is already changing the world as you read these words. Choosing the twenty-one people you will hug is an important part of the journey, because you must take the time to identify those with whom you feel close, those you want to be closer to, and those you want to connect with. You are increasing their awareness by bringing the hug into their world in a way that can inspire them. One of the beautiful things about the hug is that you can't give one without getting one. I strongly encourage you to invite your friends and family to begin their personal twenty-one-day journeys and "hug it forward." It's amazing how much love you can spread that way.

Record your journey with video clips, so that hugging it forward and the momentum of the movement occurs both organically, and through the power of the Internet. Take action in the moment and utilize your smartphone to post on Facebook, Instagram, your blog, or any place that will reach the people you care about, and also those you don't know you care about yet. The goal of the #21DAYHUG is for it to become a phenomenon that powerfully connects people around the globe.

More about social media: I was somewhat skeptical about social media at first, but then it occurred to me: Facebook and social media in general is like the Force in Star Wars. It can be used for good or evil. As a therapist, I largely stayed away from it, because it didn't seem appropriate for clients to have a view into my personal life. From my training, it just didn't feel right. Now, as a therapeutic coach, I feel freer, and have let go of some of the constraints that were holding me back. As a therapist, my other concern about Facebook is that for someone who is feeling down, it could be depressing to see everyone else posting such happy moments—getting engaged, going on an amazing vacation, having the cutest kid or animal pics, and the like. Some research has shown that having this kind of contact online can make someone who is sad feel even worse.[7]

However, embracing social media can have very nurturing and positive impacts too. I went from having about fifty friends to well over one thousand friends in just a few days. Granted, many of those connections are superficial, or in name only, but a few are much more meaningful.

When I created the twenty-one-day hug-it-forward journey, I wanted to reach people, depressed or not, and invite them to be more connected with friends and family, instead of letting them isolate themselves. The goal was to activate a whole group of people who could reach out in their tight-knit communities and around the world. This is a powerful platform for good. I want each of you to think about that moving forward as well. Facebook and social media can be hugs in and of themselves—ways to reach out to someone in any part of the world, and wrap them in a warm and cozy embrace that shares the joy of being human and

---

7   Chowdhry, Amit. "Research Links Heavy Facebook And Social Media Usage To Depression." Forbes. April 30, 2016. http://www.forbes.com/sites/amitchowdhry/2016/04/30/study-links-heavy-facebook-and-social-media-usage-to-depression/#7e7071287e4b.

Hug Therapy

connected to other people. I can only imagine what the virtual future holds.

The journey begins with your commitment to having longer hugs and even (if you chose to take it on) to hug the people in your life for twenty-one seconds for twenty-one consecutive days. This will embolden you to express your feelings for them in ways that are genuine and unique to the person you are hugging. As you take this journey, you're choosing to slow down and be present in your life as often as you possibly can. You will achieve this increased awareness by engaging in long, loving hugs that last for at least twenty-one seconds. There are many physiological benefits with twenty-one-second hugs. Equally important, a hug makes a powerful statement of love, by expressing how much the people in your life mean to you.

WHY THIS MATTERS

If you are on this journey, you have already begun to get in touch with your own music and become more attuned to your own soundtrack. Once you begin to hear your music, the challenge and the choice in each moment is if you choose to dance.

As this deepens, you will be in a state of "flow," a term coined by Mihály Csíkszentmihályi, who described it as, "being completely involved in an activity for its own sake. In flow, the ego falls away. Time flies. Every action, movement, and thought follows inevitably from the previous one, like playing jazz. Your whole being is involved, and you're using your skills to their utmost potential."[8] Don't expect to be in flow all the time. The overactive-survival mechanism is built in antiflow. When you wield supercharged mindfulness, radical transparency, and the power of the hug, you become fully responsible for your life.

The challenge is to listen deeply enough to yourself to be able to hear your music. It may be fast or slow, upbeat or melancholy. Trust that it is always playing, and that hearing it is magical. Once you begin to hear your music, the challenge and the value is to choose whether you want to dance.

If you dance to the music you hear, others might think you are crazy, but that's only because they can't hear your music. There may be times or places when you choose not to dance to your music, but in these moments, you will still be grounded and peaceful.

---

8   Csikszentmihalyi, Mihaly. *Flow: The Psychology of Optimal Experience*. New York: Harper Perennial Modern Classics, 2009.

Authenticity requires being in touch with who you are, being okay with who you are, and being who you are, even in a public place. You love who you are. You embrace who you are.

Hug Therapy is about bucking cultural norms. If you have a reason to follow a cultural norm, that's okay, but have the freedom to make a conscious choice. For example, let's say I'm ice skating or cross-country skiing around the airport in my socks. Just imagine me, shoes in hand, sliding around the airport, caught up in how it feels to slide and play. Those who notice me may be a bit surprised, or even look at me like I've lost it. Now imagine that a plane crashes into the airport and I die. Game over. Do we really have enough people embracing their inner kid and sliding through the airport in their socks? I'm advocating for you to live those few minutes as if that's all the time there is, because it may be. I'm not going to regret slipping around the airport in my socks, or playing ball with my son, even if the bouncing ball might annoy the people around us.

It doesn't serve any of us, nor the world, to operate inside a tiny box. We can be much freer, and most people won't notice or care. Those who find offense might be upset no matter what you do, because they think the world is against them or are potentially having a bad day completely unrelated to your self-expression.

We often live in prisons of our own making, but we can have more fun, and be much livelier than we realize. Most people don't care what we do. You could skip everywhere you go for twenty-one weeks, and in twenty-one days of skipping, you might get twenty-one comments, while a thousand people haven't even noticed.

We're all concerned about what is expected of us in certain settings, and what people think when we do something out of the ordinary. This book is about freedom to live your life the way you want—living your life like nobody's looking. It's about being metaphorically naked. It's about taking your shirt off. It's about being vulnerable. Why am I doing whatever I'm doing? Because I feel like it. Because my inner child wants to come out and play.

The only reason you are not free is because your overly active survival instinct is kicking in. This all goes back to survival. Survival says I should behave a certain way—I should sit a certain way, talk a certain way, act a certain way, etc., because then I will be accepted by the person over there, whom I don't even know. I'm not going to take off my shoes and socks at the airport, because it is not socially acceptable.

ACTION

Step outside of your comfort zone and step boldly with love in your heart into the "hugging zone." Share more openly with the people around you, and do the things you want to do—even if they aren't "normal" or socially acceptable (to be clear, I am not advocating anything dangerous or illegal).

Embrace who you are, and what you truly want—that is the first step in creating it.

Conclusion

Hug Therapy has presented new and valuable ways to think about and understand awareness and connection. I have worked to provide hugging guidelines to enhance your understanding of communication, relationship building, personal growth and stepping outside your "comfort zone" into the "hugging zone." The twenty-one-second hug and 21-Day Hugging Journey are based on proven physiological and psychological benefits. The combination of these benefits allows for increased happiness, effectiveness, and a profound sense of who you are in the world.

With strangers, you can develop deeply meaningful connections. This will both enrich your life in unexpected ways, and have a major impact in, and on, the world. You are invited to share these stories openly and proudly.

Go to www.thehugdoctor.com to share your journey around the world and inspire others to take it on. As mentioned, you can also powerfully share the twenty-one-day journey via Facebook Live. This allows you to leave an imprint on the world, and emboldens you to step into the hugging zone internationally. This is one of many ways to be a leader in the moment, giving a unique and beautiful touchpoint that models living, loving, and sharing, which can be deeply meaningful for your friends, family, and beyond. What will you create by both getting lost in, and living in, the space of a hug? There are a million and one ways to go on this journey. Whatever you choose, begin today. If you are not planning to start today, take a hard look at why. You can only start anything today, and if not now, when?

Start right where you are today, and begin to build momentum. Wherever you engage this journey, you are an inspiration, and this is it. There is no time like the present.

When you enter a room and think, "*Who in this room would like a hug?*" consider this is a distinct shift from what you were thinking before you embraced the hugging paradigm.

By hugging our way through the world, we not only transform our experience of the world; we transform the world itself. There really are no strangers.

Now, get out there and hug.

Why I Wrote *Hug Therapy*

In writing *Hug Therapy* I didn't have a choice and it simply came through me. The ongoing editing process has been a complex and demanding labor of love. In this section, my goal is to convey how crazy and beautiful the world is, and how we can use the hug as a tool to ground us and make the very best of our life.

It has truly been my honor and joy to share with you what really makes hugs tick, and I hope that however you take it on it will enrich your life in a multitude of ways. Now I want to point to some of the challenges we are currently facing in the world. I know in my heart that hugging tools can play a powerful role in dealing with them. One 21-second hug at a time.

When I do psychological testing, one of the questions asked is, "What does the expression 'the grass is always greener on the other side' mean to you?" Living life assuming others have it better can be a very limiting mindset. Getting overly focused on all the things that are wrong in the world is another trap. It is important to recognize these issues without becoming overwhelmed. The goals of seeing the world through the lens of a hug are to discover new ways to create a healthy outlook on life, and have access to take the actions that really matter.

Many of the things that aren't working in our world can be powerfully impacted by hugging and the hugging perspective. My purpose here is to briefly highlight the problems these issues present, to begin bringing us together on a global scale to deal with them. When we each take the hugging steps most meaningful to us, we are on the pathway to a more united and connected world.

Science and technology race forward, and new ideas and inventions are constantly being created, giving us the potential to learn, relax, and enjoy life. Advances in communication could enable us to understand and care about others as never before. However, these same remarkable advances bring rapid changes that may threaten the very fabric of who we are and the quality of our lives.

Our technological "know-how" is extraordinary. Each one of the "bajillion" cell phones used by children and grownups alike is a computer more powerful than the one that got us to the moon. Our medical capabilities make possible the replacement and repair of body parts that only years ago were science fiction. (How many people do you know or know of that have a new hip, knee, or heart?) We have technology with satellites above us providing instantaneous global communication. Social media is alluring, constantly changing, and pulling at our time and energy. Cars without human drivers are on our roads, and drones and robots are flexing their muscles.

It seems the pace of life is accelerating at an alarming rate and keeps moving faster and faster. The result can leave us feeling destabilized, as if the ground beneath us is moving unpredictably. We are strapped in on a roller coaster ride of sorts that at certain times may feel thrilling and inspiring, and at others, scary and confusing.

As we do our best to hold on and "enjoy the ride," it is even more important to have common ground with others, and appreciation of different perspectives. When we feel overwhelmed and pushed toward survival mode, the ability to relate to others can be diminished, putting us in the limiting mindset of "you are either with me or against me."

As knowledge and technology grow and the world shrinks, we may feel less in control of our everyday lives to the extent we withdraw to protect ourselves. This can lead to a downward spiral of feeling detached and lonely. In the UK, a comprehensive study was done on the issue of loneliness, and many would say we are experiencing a loneliness epidemic.

In some ways, feeling powerless isn't surprising as we learn of terrorist attacks all over the world and as acts of violence become more and more common in our own schools, places of worship, and where we go to be entertained.

Our phones and electronic devices are now being targeted with increasing frequency and sophistication, which can result in everything ranging from annoyance to identify theft. Our children "safe" at home are much more vulnerable to fall victim to online bullying or other threats tied to their connections on social media or in the ever-prevalent online gaming communities.

As we feel more vulnerable, we each deal with this lack of stability in our own way to regain a sense of control. When people feel they have no other way to handle their pain and feel completely hopeless, suicide can seem like the only option.

According to the Centers for Disease Control's National Center for Health Statistics, in 2014, in the United States, there were 42,773 reported suicides. Over 40,000 in the United States alone. On average, adjusted for age, they reported the annual US suicide rate increased 24 percent over the fifteen previous years (1999 to 2014), from 10.5 to 13.0 suicides per 100,000 people, the highest rate recorded in twenty-eight years. Their most recent data for 2016 shows the numbers continue to rise.

This doesn't take into account the millions who have struggled with depression or mental health issues and had suicidal thoughts, and either not attempted suicide or not completed suicide. I personally have felt the grips of depression and looked at everything through a dark and seemingly hopeless lens. Although I have not attempted suicide, I can definitely relate to so many who have wished they wouldn't wake up, felt they didn't care about life, and felt there was no reason to go on. These dark days, weeks, months, and years are something that so many people struggle with that it is extremely difficult to calculate the numbers.

Let's stay with the actual suicide rates for a moment. It is often hard to fathom these kinds of numbers. I grew up in a moderate to small sized coal mining town in Gillette, Wyoming. While growing up, my town had a population of about sixteen thousand people. It wasn't tiny by any means. We had one high school, and my graduating class was about four hundred students. To appreciate the magnitude of suicide in our country, consider that in 2014 alone, more than double the size of my hometown committed suicide, every man, woman, and child. What the f*ck is going on?

Suicide is dark and ugly, and something very difficult to prevent. We have many "therapeutic soldiers" doing their best to help people with medication and therapy. The research suggests, that the combination of both may be the most effective, but what is going on? It seems that despite our best efforts, we keep losing too many friends and loved ones. When I began to realize the power of hugging on all levels, it crystalized for me that this was one powerful tool to impact these sobering statistics. I believe that self-hugs (taking care of oneself), relational hugs, and coming together are essential, and perhaps more important now than ever.

This book, movement, and technology, if you will, is not designed to replace traditional therapies. This technology can help give us permission to be honest with ourselves and those around us. It can allow us to stop hiding or fooling ourselves, and get clarity about what we want to create. Too often, we and our loved ones suffer in silence. Please embrace *Hug Therapy*, and take a hard *and loving* look at your life. It is intended to be used as a tool to help us act powerfully in a way that inspires. The objective is to start in our own immediate lives, and then take the power of hugging out into the world.

Consider for a moment what is happening on a global scale. If we measure the health of the planet by the quality of its inhabitants' relationships, Earth is sick. Not a day goes by without a horrific headline about a mass murder somewhere in the world. There seems to be no antidote for the hatred and violence we see played out on our TV screens every night.

Hug Therapy offered a unique vantage point. The hug is something everyone is familiar with and yet the "space of a hug" is rich in so many ways. The hug can take you on a personal and deeply meaningful journey, allowing increased satisfaction in any domain of life you choose to focus. *Hug Therapy* dissected the hug and looked at the power of hugging comprehensively. Together we explored the entire hugging continuum from hugging that involves no physical contact to some of the longest, most connective hugs ever. The hug this book proposed is universal, and it is as much a methodology as an overt expression or action. *Hug Therapy* is invested in the reader being intentional, heartfelt, and fully engaged. The hug and hugging technology have the power to communicate affection and warmth, and to create a much deeper connection with oneself and the world— as well as cool unexpected results that emerge when we embrace humanity.

Was it audacious to suggest that the hugging technology is powerful enough to stamp out war and terror and cruelty? Yes, of course. But *Hug Therapy* is not advocating one hug or even a million hugs. It is calling for a paradigm shift, a new worldview, in which relationships are newly seen through the lens of hugging.

The word and the act have many meanings: love, kindness, compassion, caring, concern, empathy, and much more. The power of one purposeful hug is that it often leads to another and another and another, until there is a tipping point—a critical juncture at which a significant and often unstoppable change takes place—in the way humans interact with each other and themselves. I want to be around to experience that tipping point and will give out as many hugs as I can to my last breath and continue joyfully forward, spreading the profound power of hugs—I couldn't be more thrilled that we are moving forward together on this journey. Thank you so much for joining the hugging movement and from the bottom of my heart I am sending you, dear reader, the biggest of virtual hugs with lightness, freedom, and a splash of golden sunshine.

Afterword

This exciting, funny, and at times outrageous book reminds us of the Zen master's admonition to "live each day as if your hair were on fire." *Hug Therapy* is an homage to joyful, spontaneous living. It is about shedding inhibition, self-doubt, and fear, and living life as if no one's watching, judging, or criticizing you. The book's author, Stone Kraushaar—or "the Hug Doctor," as he is affectionately known—is a clinical psychologist and therapeutic coach. He encourages us to step out of our restricted, automatic existence, to take chances, to jump into daring, authentic action—action that makes us feel alive—and to encourage the people around us to do the same.

I am often drawn to the words of author and teacher Martha Beck, who writes, "Basic human contact—the meeting of eyes, the exchanging of words—is to the psyche what oxygen is to the brain. If you're feeling abandoned by the world, interact with anyone you can."[9] I have spent a large part of my life studying and teaching people how to connect with each other. I've written how understanding and accepting the

---

9 Beck, Martha. "The Lonely Season." Oprah.com. February 15, 2005. http://www.oprah.com/spirit/martha-beck-the-lonely-season.

Hug Therapy

differences in people changes the way we interact, and establishes effective, life enhancing relationships.

In reading *Hug Therapy*, I've learned a bold new way of connecting with people that takes a leap of faith and love. It asks us to accept that we all yearn for, contact—a hug, if you will—and at a deep level, we are simply waiting for the invitation.

There are many self-improvement books that encourage us to be more open and loving, but *Hug Therapy* gives us an actual technique and challenges us to turn our lives into opportunities to connect with ourselves and others. The 21-Day Journey—hugging twenty-one people in twenty-one days for twenty-one seconds—suggests that we leave our comfort zone, and embrace a life of loving others and building community.

There is scientific evidence that a twenty-one-second hug makes both the hugger and huggee feel a lot better. It releases the chemical oxytocin (also known as the hug hormone, the cuddle chemical, and the bliss hormone) into our blood system. Oxytocin plays a role in relieving depression, opening our hearts, and making us more receptive to relationships.

Don't take this small, happy book too lightly, because beneath its urging to make new friends and its coaching to live more authentic lives, lies a deep belief in the goodness and oneness of all people. The information in this book is founded on a sort of "positive psychology" on steroids. It professes, without restraint or embarrassment, that people are perfect as they are, and that the encouragement we need for our best self to blossom is a hug—an expression of trust, love, and acceptance from others.

In a time when our government, politicians, and the news media try to sell us on racial, ethnic, religious, and gender differences, *Hug Therapy* inspires us to slow down and embrace our fellow human beings, either physically or virtually, by making an emotional and spiritual connection.

I urge you to fully embrace "*Hug Therapy.*" Take up the 21-Day Journey and join the global Hugging Strangers Movement; your heart, your new friends, your community, and the world will thank you.

ROBERT TALLON
Author of *The Enneagram Connection*
and coauthor of *Awareness to Action*
St. Louis

Appendix

An excerpt from the upcoming book Peace Train *by Matt Goodman*:

Peace Train tells the extraordinary tale of how the smile and hug united to create peace on earth.

Chief Smile Officer, Matt:

When I met Stone in the early winter morning at a local coffee shop in St. Louis, my whole soul needed nourishment. It was *demanding* it! I had been through a lot in the preceding few weeks. My eighty-one-year-old best friend and smile partner, Lois, had just kicked me out of her house once again (we'll get to that saga later), and I was currently sleeping in the basement of my good friend Ben Burke's house, without a true home for the half-dozenth time in my life.

Living on the razor's edge of homelessness and poverty had become status quo for me. I had an established pedigree of coming oh-so-close to success, and then being coldly knocked down by the harsh winds of reality. As much as I possessed an optimistic attitude—after all, my job title was Chief Smile Officer—this morning I needed something even more than that. The smiles, and all the thousands of sunny-yellow happy-face stickers in my duffel bag were not working!

The night before, a mutual friend, Robyn Rosenberger, had connected Stone and me via email. Robyn was the founder and CEO of Tiny Superheroes, a wonderful organization that made superhero capes for children with disabilities and illness. It was a quick introduction, but it left me intrigued right away.

Hi Matt!

Sorry I have been out of touch…I'm trying to catch up on email…seems kind of daunting! But, most importantly, I want to introduce you to Stone. You're changing the world with smiles…he's changing the world with hugs. The two of you should DEFINITELY connect—if not the three of us together.

And I'd be happy to join!

Robyn

"You're changing the world with smiles…he's changing the world with hugs." That was the line that got me! Robyn, a superhero in her own right, had declared what I had known for a long time. My mission on earth was *big*: to change it.

You see, I was the Smile Man to his Hug Man. I had researched the medical benefits of smiling as passionately as he had researched the medical benefits of a warm, huggy embrace. And just like Stone, I was heretical in my mission of proving it. I had already stuck over forty thousand smile stickers across the country with my smile partner, Lois. And I was just getting started. *What if we combined forces,* I thought?

After reading the email, I checked out the Hug Doctor's website and watched a video of him going around Cuba, hugging strangers without a second thought. He had energy, enthusiasm, and boundless passion. And he was fearless. He explained how after twenty-one seconds, your brain releases the natural chemical oxytocin, the love drug, and that it has all sorts of amazing medical benefits. I thought twenty-one seconds was kind of long and weird, but there was something about him that drew me in. He had a crazy magnetism that I recognized.

It was a nervous night of sleep as I anticipated meeting Stone the next morning. And I felt even more nervous as I walked through the door of Kaldi's coffee shop at six in the morning. I felt the weight of the world, and I was right to feel it. Peace on earth depended on the next thirty-three seconds…

About the Author

Dr. Stone Kraushaar is a clinical psychologist and therapeutic coach who discovered the transformational power of hugs, and the difference they can make for each of us individually and globally. Fondly known as "the Hug Doctor," he professes there really are no strangers—we all share a profound connection.

The Hug Doctor wants each of us to live a life full of joyful hugging that includes hugging ourselves, hugging our families, hugging our friends, and hugging the world. He teaches people how to do that literally and metaphorically. An advocate for longer, more meaningful, and inspirational hugs, he defines a hug as any positive, healthy, and connective energy that brings acceptance, healing, and peace. It is his joy to explore and teach his pioneering discoveries in his new book *Hug Therapy*.

You will catch him on 21-day hugging journeys and inspiring others about what is created together within the "space of a hug."

Dr. Stone graduated summa cum laude from the University of Denver with his BS degree and earned his master's degree and doctorate in clinical psychology at the University of Denver. His American Psychological Association (APA)-approved psychology internship was at the UCSB Student Health Services at the University of California-Santa Barbara. He completed his post-doctoral work at Yale student health services.

He lives, works, teaches, and plays in St. Louis, Missouri.

Mango Publishing, established in 2014, publishes an eclectic list of books by diverse authors—both new and established voices—on topics ranging from business, personal growth, women's empowerment, LGBTQ studies, health, and spirituality to history, popular culture, time management, decluttering, lifestyle, mental wellness, aging, and sustainable living. We were recently named 2019's #1 fastest growing independent publisher by *Publishers Weekly*. Our success is driven by our main goal, which is to publish high quality books that will entertain readers as well as make a positive difference in their lives.

Our readers are our most important resource; we value your input, suggestions, and ideas. We'd love to hear from you—after all, we are publishing books for you!

Please stay in touch with us and follow us at:

Facebook: Mango Publishing
Twitter: @MangoPublishing
Instagram: @MangoPublishing
LinkedIn: Mango Publishing
Pinterest: Mango Publishing

Sign up for our newsletter at www.mango.bz and receive a free book!

Join us on Mango's journey to reinvent publishing, one book at a time.